Even though

The
Valley *of the*
Shadow
of Cancer

I will fear no evil,
for You are with me.

Eleanor M. Bouwman

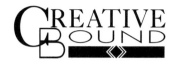

Published by Creative Bound Inc.
P.O. Box 424, Carp, Ontario
Canada K0A 1L0 (613) 831-3641

ISBN 0-921165-42-0
Printed and bound in Canada

Unless otherwise stated, all Bible quotations are taken from The New International Version, copyright © 1983 by the B.B. Kirkbride Bible Company Inc. and The Zondervan Corporation.

Book design and formatting by Wendelina O'Keefe
Front cover photo by Diarama Stock Photos Inc.

Canadian Cataloguing in Publication Program

Bouwman, Eleanor M.
      The valley of the shadow of cancer

ISBN 0-921165-42-0

      1. Bouwman, Eleanor M.   2. Cancer—Religious aspects—Christianity.   3. Cancer—Patients—Religious life.   4. Cancer—Patients—Biography.   I. Title.

RC265.6.B68A3 1996   248.8'6   C96-900080-4

Dedication

To my husband Merv,
our children David and Anita,
and the countless other people
who have faithfully approached
God's throne in prayer on my behalf
during the last six and a half years.

Acknowledgments
≈≋≈

I am eternally grateful to God for always being there, no matter how devastating the prognosis has been, and for giving me joy, peace and hope even on the darkest days, just as He has promised.

My gratitude also goes to Merv who has loved and encouraged me, prayed for me, changed his diet to fit mine, and who still rearranges his work schedule to accompany me on my very frequent visits to doctors' offices, labs, hospitals and the Cancer Clinic.

Thanks also to my children who, without complaint, have walked with me in the Valley, even though my cancer crises have had a profound impact on their lives. Special thanks to Anita for typing and helping to edit this book.

I am also grateful to those doctors, whose knowledge, expertise and special precautions, have helped me to cope with, as well as control, this disease.

Much gratitude goes to John F. Coombs, B.Sc., M.D., for always speaking life and hope and for taking time out of his very busy schedule to review this manuscript.

My gratitude also goes to David J. Klaassen, M.D., FRCPC, Vice President and Executive Director of the Vancouver Cancer Center for reading my manuscript and writing a review.

I give my thanks to our friends Frank and Pat, Alf and Christa, David and Dawn, Paul and Joyce, Gary and Barbara, and my sister Carolyn, for their contribution in editing.

And to all the others who continue to pray for our family as we push ahead in our battle against cancer, thank you and God bless.

Introduction

*S*ix and a half years ago, when I received the news that I had cancer, I read as much on the subject as I could. I was disappointed because I was unable to find what I was looking for. There were lots of cancer books that were purely scientific and statistical. They gave me medical information, but I wanted more. I also found books dealing with the disease using New Age concepts and Eastern Mysticism. Since these are not part of my faith, I avoided them. What I was desperately searching for was a book about the joys and fears, laughter and tears, victories and defeats, good prognoses and bad, as experienced by an ordinary Christian family. How did they cope with cancer? How did they keep their faith intact? How were the children affected? What did they learn? Did the family member with cancer survive? Did the *family* survive the ordeal?

It was several years and several crises later when my thoughts turned to organizing my notes and recollections into the form of a book. That seemed frightening as well as impossible, but I remembered how badly *I* had wanted to find a book like that. So what I have done is simply chronicled the cancer "highlights" during those years. I have included a lot of details which may seem superfluous. However, they show that battling cancer is an everyday struggle. Even the little things can become very complicated.

I have been painfully honest about our deepest emotions in dealing with this disease. No one in the family can escape its effects. In fact, many times the role of the patient is easier than that of the other family members. The days of good health and negative test results need to be celebrated, because no one knows the time of the next crisis. The anger, disappointments and frustrations need to be dealt with. I remember the day when Anita said, "Mom, all you ever talk about is cancer." She was right; I needed to be told.

I felt strongly that a family picture should be included, since this is a story about our family. We had many "posed" pictures, but our friends encouraged us to use the silly one you'll find on the back cover. They thought it best demonstrated that even in the face of a death sentence, we have chosen to enjoy life.

For the last three years my condition has been treated as terminal. However, not only have I survived, I feel perfectly healthy. I believe this is due to a combination of prayer, God's grace, excellent doctors, optimum nutrition, vitamins and supplements, a good sense of humor, and my conviction that I must live every day to the fullest, leaving the final outcome in the hands of my loving Heavenly Father.

It is my prayer that as you read the extraordinary events in this very ordinary family's life, you will learn from our struggles and successes, weaknesses and strengths, and thereby become better equipped to continue *your* journey with *your* family in the Valley of the Shadow of Cancer.

~ 1 ~

*I*t was a cold, dark Ottawa Valley winter morning that greeted me as I left my warm bed early on February 21, 1989. As usual, I spent the first hour of my day in the prayer room of the retreat house where my husband Merv and I and our two children lived. On that particular morning I had my seventy-nine-year-old dad on my mind. He was scheduled for surgery in a few hours for the removal of several bladder stones. I prayed for his safety and I also thanked God that none of his tests had revealed any malignancy. The whole family was concerned about that because many of his uncles and cousins had died of cancer. After my quiet time with the Lord, I went into the kitchen and peered out into the darkness to check the weather. It was a bit blustery and I hoped it would clear, as I had my yearly mammogram that afternoon in Ottawa and I didn't like winter driving at the best of times. Cancer is also prevalent in my mother's family. She had suffered from breast cancer a few years earlier. Because of this, from the age of forty, I had been advised to have a yearly mammogram. So at age forty-five, this was my fifth one. I did not consider it a big deal.

After a hurried breakfast my husband kissed me good-bye and left for work. Soon Anita, whose fourteenth birthday we had celebrated a week earlier, and David, who was seventeen, were ready to meet the school bus. As I said good-bye I reminded them to pray for Grandpa during the day. I usually watched them walk out our long country lane to see if the bus was on time. If it was late, I would drive out and the kids could wait in the warmth of the car. But that morning as I watched I began to sense that something was not quite right, for very suddenly I began to feel as if I was getting the flu. Soon the glow of the bus headlights shone through the early morning gloom onto the snow-covered road and I turned away to do my kitchen chores. When I finished I felt quite ill, with pain developing in the front and back of my abdomen.

By nine o'clock there was still a lot of blowing snow and I felt too sick to drive to Ottawa. I was happy to have an excuse to cancel the mammogram. I would not have to battle the bad weather after all. Soon the pain began to intensify very rapidly. I phoned Merv to ask him to come home immediately to take me to the doctor. He was out of the office, but the secretary, sensing my urgency, promised to contact him as soon as possible. I needed to use the washroom, and was shocked to see that the urine I had passed was pink. The pain continued to increase. Fearing I would faint, I phoned my neighbor, Nancy, who is a nurse. She came promptly. I began vomiting and rolling on the floor in excruciating pain.

Merv phoned to say that he was on the way, and arrived home in record time. Then I made a decision that proved to be wrong, perhaps even deadly, but since I had asked God to care for us during that day I somehow feel it was all in His plan. I decided that instead of going to a doctor in the city, I should go to the small town hospital only a few kilometers away. I sensed that in my condition I would be needing hospital care. As we drove off, I clutched a four pound margarine tub to use as a 'barf bucket.'

I could hardly walk up the stairs at the hospital, but somehow Merv got me in. I was bent in a ninety degree angle and was immediately ushered into an examining room. I told the nurse that the pain was much worse than labor, and she guessed that I had a kidney stone. Since she had also had one, she understood what I was experiencing. The pain was so extreme that I paced the floor, rocked from side to side, and sometimes rested my upper body on the examining table while my feet still "walked." A doctor entered and tried to examine me while I continued to move constantly. This non-stop motion embarrassed me, so I asked him why I just *had* to move. He replied, "You're diagnosing your own illness. Your symptoms, including the moving, are classic textbook symptoms of kidney stones, which is the worst pain known to man." I was relieved to know that he realized the intensity of my pain. He gave me a shot of Demerol and said that I would be fine in about twenty minutes, and then I could go home. When he returned to say good-bye, he was very surprised to see me in the same condition as when he had left me half an hour before. It was very easy for him to give me the second Demerol in the hip, as I was still bent over. Then I was taken to the radiology department. There, with every nerve in my body screaming "MOVE! MOVE! MOVE!" I had to lie still enough for the technician to take the x-ray. That was next to impossible. The x-ray did not locate the kidney stone.

The second Demerol had no effect either. I was admitted as a hospital patient, and a fast IV drip was started to quickly flush the stone out of my system. Sometime later I was given a third shot of Demerol. I rolled back and forth in bed, saying, "Jesus, where are You?" sometimes audibly and sometimes under my breath. Never having experienced agony like that, I felt abandoned. I have since learned that He is indeed there, no matter how great the suffering.

At times my thoughts and prayers were with my father, and in spite of the pain, I found it quite humorous that urinary stones had hospitalized both of us that day. What a coincidence! At 3:30 p.m. the Demerol finally took effect. Praise the Lord!

I asked Merv to go home to be there when the kids arrived from school. Being a stay-at-home Mom, I was usually there when they came home. If I wasn't, I always left a note telling them where I was. Since writing a note had not been high on my list of priorities when I had left for the hospital that morning, I wanted him to be there.

At suppertime I sat on the edge of my bed and picked at my food. My head, which felt about a foot higher than the rest of my body, seemed to spin as the Demerol traveled through my system.

Merv and the kids visited me after supper. I lay there laughing and telling them how weird I had acted, and I assured them that I would be home the following morning. We had a great time. David and Anita left to go to the Youth Group at our church, and Merv stayed with me.

Before Merv left, I buzzed the nurse to help me get to the washroom because I was still very dizzy when I stood up. Because it was expected that I would pass a kidney stone, I had to urinate into a special basin. The nurse and I checked what I had passed. Instead of seeing urine with a kidney stone in it, we saw liquid that appeared dark red, almost black. It looked like pure blood with clots in it. Fear gripped my heart. The nurse walked away with it, hardly saying a word, but her body language showed that her shock was no less than mine. I went back to bed and told Merv. We tried to encourage each other, but an icy coldness settled in our hearts.

The doctor came to see me before he went home for the night. When I told him about the urine, he said, "Ohh…" in a way that frightened me. I asked if that was normal for a kidney stone, and he said that it could be. He told me that he would discharge me the next morning after I had an ultrasound. He wanted to try again to locate the stone. We were encouraged that I could still go home as planned.

We arranged for a friend to pick me up, as Merv's schedule the next day was very full. Merv and I prayed before he left for home.

My spirits lifted as I lay in the semi-darkness. I thanked God that the horrible pain was gone, and that I was able to go home. I asked Him to heal whatever needed healing, for myself and my father. I prayed for the kids' safety, as they still had a long drive back from Ottawa, and David had not done much night driving since getting his license.

During the night I passed more blood, and again I went back to bed with a troubled heart. God was gracious and granted me sleep.

The next morning was a wonderful, crisp, sunny day. I was in good spirits. The urine I had just passed was barely pink, and I would be on my way home shortly. I rejoiced that I could lie still for the ultrasound. The pain was totally gone, so there was no need to move.

Just before I left the hospital the doctor told me to drink lots of water to prevent the development of more kidney stones. I was prepared to drink a gallon of water a day if it would spare me from ever experiencing that kind of agony again. I was also told to strain my urine for a week and bring the stone for analysis if I found it.

My friend arrived and we laughed all the way home. I told her how I had acted, and she told some stories of her own from when she had been a nurse on the urology floor. Apparently kidney stones are notorious for causing bizarre behavior.

It was wonderful to be home. I was fine and my father was recovering nicely after his surgery. The pain and drugs left me quite exhausted, so the next few days were quiet. I enjoyed the tranquillity and beauty of the winter woods beside our house. Life was good and we thanked God for His blessings. Little did we know that our family had taken its first steps into the Valley of the Shadow of Cancer.

🙦 2 🙤

March arrived and with it came one of my favorite times of the year. Each year at this time we made preparations for boiling maple syrup and I loved every minute of it, in spite of the extra work. The retreat property consisted of some cleared land, a cedar bush and a maple bush. Many people from the church had donated money to build and equip the new sugar house that Merv had designed. The syrup was sold to generate funds for the maintenance of the retreat house and property. It was a good source of extra income and it was fun. The sap usually started running around the middle of March, so volunteers came to clean the equipment, drill the trees and hang the buckets. Eventually everything was ready and I could almost smell the maple flavored smoke and steam that would soon be flowing from the vents at the top of the sugar house.

As spring pushed back winter, the days became warmer and the sap began to run. On a good day, when the sap was running quickly, the buckets had to be emptied frequently. It took over an hour to empty all of them. Therefore, when the sap had been collected from the last buckets, the first had collected an inch or two of fresh sap. The sound of the sap dripping into the empty buckets was amazing. I would stand in the middle of the bush and marvel at this wonderful music. The sound each drip produced had its own pitch, depending on the depth of sap.

I kept the workers supplied with fresh muffins and coffee. Several times a day I would taste the syrup straight from the boiler, and quickly learned to let the spoon and syrup cool before putting it into my mouth! As I did most of the bottling, I knew that if the syrup was not thick enough I would have to boil it for a bit on the kitchen stove. So I always jokingly bugged the guys to, "Boil it a few more minutes."

We all had a good time, and lots of fun and camaraderie took place. The kidney stone episode was in the past and life was continuing as usual.

※※

On March 29, five weeks after being discharged from the hospital, I received a phone call from a doctor in Ottawa. I was told that I should come in for an appointment as a follow-up to my stay in the hospital. That surprised me. I asked if there was a problem, and was assured there wasn't. As we were in the midst of all the maple syrup work, and since there was no problem, it was decided that I would see that doctor the following week.

The next week the doctor showed me a letter he had just received from the hospital, reporting that they had not found a kidney stone. Instead, the ultrasound had revealed a ten-centimeter (four-inch) hypernephroma on my left kidney. They felt it should be investigated further. The letter was very casual, so I was not alarmed. I asked the doctor what a hypernephroma was, and he admitted that he did not know. He also said he would make an appointment with a urologist. When I wondered what that specialist would do, the doctor replied that he wasn't sure as he had never had a patient with that diagnosis. Before I left, he said that the one thing he did know about a hypernephroma was that it is never cancer. That was all I needed to hear to dispel any apprehension I had felt. After all, if it was something serious the hospital would not have waited five weeks to inform the doctor, right?

On the way home I stopped at Nancy's house to pick up a nursing textbook. Hypernephroma was not in it. I asked another friend who is a nurse and she didn't know either, so we just forgot about it.

The appointment with the urologist was set up for May 12—another five and a half weeks away. The next day I told one of the maple syrup helpers about my upcoming appointment with the urologist. That doctor had been his surgeon, and he told me he was an excellent doctor as well as a Christian. I was delighted!

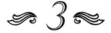

Maple syrup time was coming to an end. Spring was definitely in the air, and most nights were too warm to drive the sap down to the tree roots. That was necessary for its flow the next day. With a little help from my imagination, I could see tiny buds developing on the canopy of maple branches high overhead.

The following week, while Robin was boiling the last batch of syrup, I told him about my kidney stone saga. He became very serious as I spoke. His concern was well founded because he had had two kidney transplants. He knew all about kidney problems.

It was dusk when I left the sugar house. The moon was shining brilliantly in the dark blue sky. The mud squished under my rubber boots as I made my way to the house. I breathed deeply, enjoying the warm spring air. It was then that I had a thought that I believe was inspired by the Holy Spirit. Perhaps Robin would have a urology book, and I could read up on hypernephroma before seeing the urologist. I went back into the warm, steamy sugar house. He said yes, he did have a book on the subject; he would bring it two days later when he was coming out again to help transplant several dozen maple saplings. Since our trees were old, we had decided to expand the bush for future use.

Two days later, at about five o'clock in the afternoon, the cars began to arrive for the planting bee. I had made a big pot of soup for the workers, and as I was stirring it I watched for Robin's car. I eagerly anticipated learning about my condition. He finally arrived and came into the kitchen with the book. I was delighted and continued stirring the soup as I said, "Great! You remembered to bring the book!" I looked up and saw that he was not nearly as enthusiastic as I was. He said he was not sure he should give the book to me. In fact, the only condition under which he would let me read it was that I would have to take into consideration that the book was twenty years old, and according to it, he should be dead by now. I continued stirring (I couldn't feed twenty men burnt soup!) and asked, "Is it that bad?" Robin answered, "Yes," handed me the book and left the kitchen. I opened it to the page he had marked, and while still stirring, I read that eighty per cent of hypernephromas are malignant and the treatment is always removal of the kidney. There was other bad news as well, but maybe I was in the other twenty per cent. After all, I was feeling perfectly healthy, the book was twenty years old, and I had to set the table. I quickly prayed for peace as I prepared to feed the workers.

Later that evening when the last tree planter left, I handed the book to Merv and shared the news with him. We prayed and once again tried to be strong for each other. Since this was Friday night we could not contact the doctor until Monday. Needless to say it was a very heavy weekend. We decided not to tell the kids anything at all until we knew more ourselves.

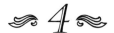

*E*arly Monday morning I phoned the doctor in Ottawa. I was told to phone the urologist and ask for the first appointment cancellation because the one scheduled was still several weeks away. I did that. The next morning I was informed that an ultrasound was booked for Friday.

The nurse also said that in order to speed things up, the urologist wanted to talk to me immediately on the phone instead of waiting for an appointment. He asked the regular questions: weight, height, family members, a description of what had taken place eight weeks before at the hospital, and how I was feeling now. He informed me that it would take several days to get the results of the ultrasound and that he was going to be out of town until the following Wednesday. On Thursday he would let me know the results. He was horrified that so much time had been lost since the initial symptoms had appeared. I began to grasp the fact that I might not be in the other twenty per cent after all. During the next eight days I did much praying and Bible reading. We asked our close friends to intercede for us. I asked for peace and God gave it.

One morning during my prayer time, I realized that I needed to forgive the doctor at the hospital as well as the Ottawa doctor for the loss of many weeks of precious time. Why did that hospital wait five weeks to inform the doctor in Ottawa? Why didn't the radiologist who discovered the ten-centimeter mass treat it as an emergency? Why did the Ottawa doctor tell me that hypernephroma is never cancer? I knew that somehow I needed to forgive them. I very rarely have prostrated myself on the floor before the Lord, but that morning I did. I forgave the erring doctors as well as I could—even if their errors could cause my death. When I finally stood up I had no anger or bitterness left. I knew that if I died, I could face Jesus with no unforgiveness in my heart.

As I continued to read the scriptures, I was hoping to find all the healing verses because I do believe in miracles. Those passages did not mean much to me at that time. Instead my comfort came from the Psalms, especially Ps. 73:23-26.

Yet I am always with you; you hold me by my right

hand. You guide me with your counsel, and afterward you will take me into glory. Whom have I in heaven but you? And being with you, I desire nothing on earth. My flesh and my heart may fail, but God is the strength of my heart and my portion forever.

That surely was not about healing, but it ministered to me immensely.

≈∂≈

I wondered how I should pray about my situation. Eventually I got to the point where I could say this prayer: "Lord I believe You can heal me. If that is Your will I would thank You and give You the glory. But if surgery would bring You more glory, I am willing to go to the hospital. If my death could bring You the most glory, I am willing." It took me a while to be able to say that last part.

≈∂≈

The next Thursday morning, I stayed close to the phone. Finally around eleven o'clock, the urologist phoned. This call was one of the most memorable I have ever received. He confirmed that I had a solid mass on my left kidney and that I was booked into the hospital the following Wednesday. He would meet me there that evening. He sounded very concerned and asked if I had any questions. I wanted him to be more specific about the solid mass, but he said he could not tell me anything more at that time. I told him that God had prepared me for the worst, and that I had peace. He asked me if I knew the Lord, and sounded very relieved that God was involved in this situation. He acknowledged that he also was a Christian and, therefore, knew the peace that I was experiencing. We talked about how difficult illnesses like this must be for non-believers. He ended the conversation with, "And now we'll just have to wait and see how the Lord pulls you through this."

I hung up and felt like dancing for joy. To have a surgeon who knows Jesus and His peace was a wonderful blessing.

5

*D*oes God take care of small details? Yes, He does.

I usually cooked for about three out of every four retreats, but that weekend, the retreatants were bringing their own food. That meant I would be free on Saturday. I was looking forward to the weekend. It had been lonely that week being by myself from seven in the morning until four-thirty when the kids arrived home from school. My thoughts and prayers were all centered on the tumor and what that would mean for us as a family. On Saturday there would be lots of people around and my family would be there too. I thought that would be wonderful.

On Friday night a school friend called Anita, inviting her to spend Saturday at her house. This friend had never phoned before, in fact, she and Anita had never visited each other. I had really wanted to spend time with Anita. After all, if I died, that would be our last Saturday together. I desperately wanted to tell her that she couldn't go, but somehow I felt that the Holy Spirit was telling me that she should. With great difficulty I agreed, and said I would drive her there.

The drive the next morning took almost an hour. I must admit I felt a real heaviness. I had a brief chat with her friend's mother and learned that they also are believers. I was very happy for Anita. If I died, it would be good for her to have the support of a Christian friend at school.

On the way home I cried for the first time, not for myself, but for my parents. I felt so sorry that they would have to deal with my illness from five hundred kilometers away.

When I arrived home, the house was full of people and Merv was planting trees, so I went to our private quarters.

There, surrounded by the joyful sounds of twenty retreatants, I felt very lonely. In fact, I felt very restless. I wanted to run away, but I didn't know where to run. The peace I had experienced all week was wearing thin and I was edgy all day. I even began to wonder about the urologist whom I had not met. At one point I walked the trails in the bush. Then I went to Merv and watched him plant shrubs and bushes. The thought came to me that I probably would not see them bloom the next spring. I comforted myself by imagining that the plants in heaven would be more beautiful. I looked at Merv and thought that he probably would get remarried if I died. Since we were married twenty-two years at the time and he was only forty-five, he might have a longer marriage to a second wife. That hurt, but once again I comforted myself. We had a very good relationship, but our marriage and any years of a second marriage would only be like an instant in eternity. That day is one I remember well.

❧❧

Later that afternoon Merv asked me to make him some sandwiches for supper as he still had many shrubs to plant. What happened next is an example of God's timing and grace. The very moment I walked out of the house with the sandwiches, Anita was getting out of her friend's car. I had not heard them drive in, and if I had been fifteen seconds later, the car would have left. The mother saw me, so I walked over to the car. She and her daughter got out, and the two girls, suspecting that their Moms would talk for a while, disappeared into the house. I decided to share my situation with her, warning her not to say anything in front of the girls when they returned. Our kids had not been told how serious my condition might be.

She asked who the surgeon was. When I told her, she was delighted and said that he had been a family friend for many years. She assured me that he was an excellent doctor and a very dedicated Christian. She said that I would be having the very best care available. I felt that God had arranged this conversation about my doctor whom I had not yet met. All my heaviness and anxieties completely disappeared. I knew then why it had been so important for Anita to spend the day with this family. My heart sang as I took the sandwiches to Merv. My faith and peace were intact once again. To me this was a miracle: a girlfriend's first invitation to Anita, my going out at precisely the right moment, and the mother knowing the urologist and confirming the fact that he was a Christian as well as a highly respected surgeon. Coincidence? I don't think so. It was as if God was using these events to show that He was in control.

That night I dreamt I was at the hospital meeting a new doctor. She asked me if I had forgiven the doctors who had made the mistakes. I told her that I had. Then, as we walked down the hall, we met a woman who was rolling on the floor in pain just as I had been ten weeks earlier. The doctor stopped, taught her a little Jesus song, and told her to sing it whenever the pain was unbearable. I was impressed that she was a believer, and as we continued down the hall I asked her if she believed that God can heal. She replied, "Don't you know that God always heals tumors, sometimes before we die and sometimes after?" With that I woke up. That last sentence did not reassure me that I would live, but I had overflowing peace as I went back to sleep. Unfortunately, I have never remembered the words of that little Jesus song, but I believe that the dream was from the Lord to strengthen me.

The next day at church I learned that another woman my age was scheduled for surgery that week, following the discovery of a lump in her breast. We comforted each other and promised to pray.

Later that day the next group using the retreat house facility arrived, and once again God's wisdom and timing were perfect. We often had groups during the week and I always cooked for them. It was too difficult to get the kids off to school, Merv off to work and the preparations for the next weekend retreat done, if I had to work around others in my kitchen. On the weekends when I did not cook, we moved into our living room and sort of "camped" there for the weekend, leaving the kitchen free for the retreatants. This arrangement did not work during the week. When the Campus Crusade for Christ representative made the booking months ahead, she said that they would do the meals themselves. I explained that I always provided meals during the week as that was easier for me. She persisted, saying that they would work around my kitchen schedule. Now, I was very thankful that I had agreed. I had no worries about how they would be fed. That was very important, considering I would soon be in the hospital.

I had wondered how we would sleep on my last night at home. Would fear overtake my peace? Anita had been taking a baby-sitting course and her final test was that night. We dropped her off and then went to pray with the woman who was scheduled for breast surgery. When we picked up Anita she was ecstatic. She had received the highest mark on the test and she wanted to celebrate. We found a little Chinese restaurant and there Anita, Merv and I laughed as we ate our egg rolls. We went home and all of us had a good night's sleep, enjoying Anita's success.

The next morning, May 3, 1989, just before leaving for the hospital, I phoned my parents and told them what I was facing. I had waited until then to tell them so they would not worry. My mother asked if it could be serious. I said it could. I hoped I would never have to phone them with that kind of news again. When I was ready to go, I poked my head into the lounge where the retreatants were, told them about my hospitalization, and asked for their prayers. Merv and I were very quiet as we drove out the lane. I wondered if I would ever drive *in* that lane again.

～ 6 ～

At the hospital, admission and the preliminary tests went very well, even though I had visions of getting lost. One of my friends who is a part-time nurse there was off duty that morning, so she had come especially to be my guide. She had lunch with Merv and me, and when Merv left for work, she stayed and we chatted in my hospital room about our families. The subject of cancer never came up.

That evening, I was halfway through supper when the radiologist came in and asked if the urologist had already seen me. When I said he hadn't, he made a very hasty retreat, saying that he would be back after I had seen the other doctor. In a few minutes a doctor arrived and introduced himself as the urologist. He asked a few questions about what I did at the retreat house to relieve the tension. Then he started discussing what would happen the next morning. The radiologist would embolize my kidney, which meant he would kill it. That would cause the tumor to die. In six days the urologist would remove the dead kidney and dead tumor. I asked if he couldn't remove only the tumor. He said, "The kidney has to go." I looked him in the eye and said, "Then it's cancer, isn't it?" and he replied, "Yes." I had wondered how it would feel to be told I had cancer. My sister had been with my mother when she was told that the lump in her breast was malignant. They thought the doctor had been rather blunt. So there I was, having confirmed what I had already suspected, and I felt only peace. I knew it definitely was the peace that passes all understanding (Phil. 4:7).

Still, I suggested that it might be a cyst, because an immediate family member once had a very large benign uterine cyst. Mine might also be benign. The urologist informed me that almost one hundred per cent of kidney tumors are malignant. We chatted a bit more, and then he left. I was alone. I pushed away the remainder of my supper. I had lost my appetite.

Almost immediately the radiologist returned, and he also seemed like a good friend who was there to help. He drew a diagram of a body with kidneys and arteries, and described how and why he would embolize my kidney. He would insert an instrument up the artery located where the right leg joins the body. The blood supply to the cancerous left kidney would then be blocked. This would result in the death of both the kidney and tumor. At that point, my immune system would be coping with a dead kidney and tumor, and it would jump into "overdrive," producing specialized cells to destroy renal cell cancer. I thought it sounded as though my immune system would be doing its own chemotherapy, and the doctor agreed that it was somewhat similar. He advised me that I would be heavily sedated with a very strong narcotic, Dilaudid, because the pain would be totally unbearable. I would be in the Intensive Care Unit (ICU) for six days. He stressed the importance of never letting the pain get out of control. I would have to ask for more pain killers at the first twinge of pain. I would have lots of Tylenol to control my elevated temperature, and Gravol for any nausea I might experience. I was going to be VERY ILL! Before he left, he enthusiastically said he could guarantee that after the kidney was removed on the sixth day, I would have no more living kidney cancer cells in my body. I really clung to those words!

I knew that Merv and the kids were coming to see me, but I wanted to talk to Merv first. My mind was so preoccupied with all those facts, that trying to place a long distance phone call from my hospital room was out of the question. I called a friend in the city and asked her to phone Merv to tell him to leave the kids in the lobby and come up alone. I prayed as I waited for him. When he walked into the room I began to tell him everything at once, stressing the positive aspects but also telling him of the horrendous six days that were ahead of us. We tried to be strong for each other while wondering how to tell the kids.

He went down to get them. When they returned together, I again went through what I had just learned, stressing the good parts even more while minimizing the events of the next six days. David and Anita, true to their own unique personalities, reacted to the news differently. Anita became quiet and looked straight ahead. Dave started laughing and tried to joke about having one kidney. He needed to break the tension. I was concerned for Anita and asked if she was okay. She said she was fine, but was afraid that if she would wake up in the middle of the night, she wouldn't be able to go back to sleep again. I suggested that she should awaken Merv so he could pray with her. I checked later and by God's grace she slept all night. We joined hands before they went home and Merv prayed for all of us. We were beginning to realize that when one member of a family goes through the Valley of the Shadow of Cancer, the rest of the family walks there too.

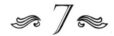

When I awoke the next morning it seemed that I had prayed and quietly sung songs of praise all night. I felt rested and began my quiet time with the Lord. I was following a back issue of the daily devotional *Every Day With Jesus*. When I finished that, I remembered that Merv had bought the current one which I had not yet started to read. I had the feeling that I should read the passage in the new booklet for that day, Thursday, May 4, 1989. Because I felt so strongly that I needed to read it, I thought there might be some encouraging words there for me. The scripture meditation for the day was 2 Cor. 1:3-14. When I opened my Bible to that passage, I couldn't believe what I saw. There were three sections underlined, and in the margin adjacent to those passages I had written the numbers 1-2-3. I quickly read the first underlined verse. It said, "...so that we can comfort those in trouble with the comfort we ourselves have received from God." That was exciting because just the night before, Merv and I had speculated that God might use me at the retreat house to bring comfort and hope to others who were facing this disease. I read the next underlined section. "But this happened that we might not rely on ourselves but on God, who raises the dead." My excitement rose as this fit too. I was certainly depending on God to raise me from this death bed. The third underlined section almost jumped off the page. "Then many will give thanks on our behalf for the gracious favor granted us in answer to the prayers of many." I had no idea when or why I had marked those verses, but I rejoiced as I let those words sink in. Deep down, I believed that I would survive the six days and the surgery, "in answer to the prayers of many." I quickly phoned a friend and told her that I thought I would live. She thanked God when I told her about the passage.

While I waited eagerly to share those scriptures with Merv, the woman in the next bed started yelling. She demanded that I pull back the curtain around my bed so she could see the sunshine too. Who was I to think that I could keep the curtain pulled and leave her in the dark? I tried to explain that I was facing cancer surgery and needed to be by myself, but she kept on complaining. When the nurse came, I asked her what I should do. She told me to leave the curtain drawn if that was what I needed. I felt sorry for that woman. I suspected that she probably did not have the prayer support nor the peace of mind that God had given me, because she had also been rude the night before.

Merv was happy to see those verses, but they did not give him the confidence they gave me. Later I walked the hall for a bit, and even though I believed those reassuring words were from the Lord, I still felt a grieving within me. The people I met smiled and greeted me, but I was very aware of the Valley of the Shadow of Cancer.

～⁓～

I have almost no recollection of how or where the embolization took place. I remember the radiologist announcing that he was starting, and I recall feeling the pressure of his thumb to close the hole which the instruments had made in my artery. He had told me about that previously, so I knew the procedure was finished. I spent the next six days in the ICU. Never having been in that part of a hospital, I imagined that it would be very quiet. Instead it was a very busy, sometimes noisy, place. The beds were separated with curtains, so sound traveled easily. As I was going to be there for many days, I was given the bed beside the window. When the plants and bouquets began to arrive, I was able to keep some on the window sill. Due to the drugs, I remember very little of those six days. I recall having a very strong craving for an Egg McMuffin. Why, I don't know, but Merv promised that when I was released, we'd go to McDonald's to get one. That craving was especially overwhelming when I saw yet another bowl of green Jell-O or a cup of broth coming toward me!

During this time I seemed to be floating in a vacuum. I knew my family, but I didn't know where they had come from or where they were going when they left. I could not process anything beyond the immediate present or outside the walls of the ICU. My window overlooked the road, and I remember watching the cars during rush hour every morning. It made absolutely no sense to me why they were there. Easy tasks became very difficult. It took all my concentration and effort to change a tape in the small tape player Merv had bought for me. Getting the earphones into my ears was quite a challenge!

The most distressing limitation was my inability to pray.

I had planned to intercede for the others in the ICU as well as for myself, but I just couldn't gather my thoughts enough to pray. One day a young girl and a young man were admitted. They both had overdosed on drugs, but I could not pray for them. I felt guilty about that and shared it with my pastor. He told me to just rest in Jesus and let others do the praying. He said I should remember the poem *Footprints*, and realize that there was only one set of footprints during that time. That comforted me.

One night I awakened shortly after midnight and thought I was hallucinating. I heard a voice in a monotone (I could not tell if it was male or female) that seemed to be telling his or her life story. After a long time, I rang for a nurse and asked if this really was happening or was I going crazy. She laughed and said there was a woman with a deep voice in the next bed, telling the story of her life to whoever would listen. I was relieved to hear that.

The only visitors allowed in the ICU were immediate family and clergy. My very close friend Margaret is only a few years younger than my mother. She came in her place, since Mom couldn't be there. Margaret came almost every day. We hardly talked. She would pat my arm and say, "It's okay, Eleanor. You don't need to talk. I'll just sit here and pray." It was wonderful to doze off knowing she was surrounding me with her prayers.

One day three pastors visited me within an hour. Two were former pastors and one was our interim pastor. Despite my confusion, I chuckled when the third arrived. I told Merv that the nurses must think I am either very spiritual or very bad to have so many clergy concerned about me.

I needed the narcotics about every five hours. My temperature was taken regularly day and night, and I was given Tylenol if it was too high. At times I was nauseated so I was given a shot of Gravol. That had a pleasant side effect—it put me to sleep. My hips were very sore and bruised from all the needles. After a few days my whole body itched. I'm not a complainer, but I finally had to tell the nurse how uncomfortable I was. The nurses were advised to provide me with bedding which had been washed in special soap. The itchiness soon left. A few days later I overheard the nurses talking about a man whose kidney had also been embolized. He was experiencing the same reaction. They concluded that this was to be expected. We were among the first in the city to undergo this procedure, so the medical staff was learning too.

On the morning of the sixth day, I awoke and realized that even though it had been much longer than five hours since I was given my last painkiller, I felt no pain. As the morning dragged on, I became fearful. Why was there no pain? What had happened inside of me? Had more of me than just the kidney and tumor died? Two nurses came in and started shaving my midsection, front and back. I was unaware that I had hair on my upper abdomen that needed shaving. While one nurse used a razor the other held a flashlight so they would not miss any of these invisible hairs. I began to wonder if I was going to be cut in half by the surgeon, considering the large area they shaved. Finally the radiologist came in. When I told him about my lack of pain, he was delighted and said, "Great! Your body is done fighting. It's time for the surgery."

As my surgery was scheduled for 5:30 p.m., the day seemed long without food or drink. At last the nurses with their strange green head and shoe covers came to get me. I had been given the "pre-op cocktail," and in my wooziness, I realized that I had to urinate. In came the bed pan and out the door went any sense of pride or privacy I had left. Merv and Margaret had prayed with me, and as I was wheeled to the operating room, they headed for the chapel to spend the time in prayer.

The next thing I knew, I was in the recovery room, feeling as though someone was trying to suffocate me. A nurse was holding an oxygen mask over my mouth and nose. I tried desperately to shove it aside, but she was even more determined to keep it in place. That was an awful experience. As I drifted in and out of consciousness, I became aware that I was in extreme pain. I begged for more painkillers, but the nurse said that I had had all that I was allowed. The pain seemed even worse than it had eleven weeks before, but they insisted I could not have anything for the pain until I returned to the ICU. I recall thinking that I felt as if a horse had kicked me just below the ribs on my left side. I have no idea why that image came to mind, but it seemed to be a good description.

I finally made the long journey from the OR on the first floor to the ICU on the fourth. I felt every irregularity in the floor, and when the wheels of the stretcher went over the gap between the elevator and the hall floor I thought my side would split open. I'm sure we must have been going slowly, but it felt as if we were racing down an expressway.

When we reached our destination I begged for a painkiller, but after looking at my chart, the nurse told me I could not have any more. I must have gone to sleep, as I remember nothing else about that night.

The next morning with the help of painkillers and an IV, the pain was gone, but was I sore! My whole left side felt like one massive bruise. Judging from the size of the bandages, I assumed that I must have a very large incision. I learned that I also had a splenectomy, and as a result was given three units of blood. Apparently my spleen had been attached to my kidney, and when the surgeon tried to separate the two organs, the spleen ruptured. This distressed me because only recently AIDS had been linked to tainted blood used in transfusions. When the kids came to visit me, all the tubes and machines freaked them out. In fact, David told me that if I didn't leave my arm with the IV under the covers, he'd pass out and need a bed too. I tried to laugh, but it hurt too much.

By the next day I was feeling quite good, although I was still very sore and exhausted. I was told I could leave the ICU and move to a semi-private room. After eight days in the ICU, that was very welcome news, but by evening there was still no bed available. The urologist knew how desperately I wanted to be in a regular room, so after a few phone calls he found one that was available. The trip to my new room was a very pleasant one.

A hematologist visited me and explained that the loss of my spleen was not serious. Other organs would eventually take over the spleen's job. To protect me from infections, I would need an injection called Pneumovax, which would be given in a few weeks. He warned me that I might be more susceptible to infections until that time. As I was not at all prone to having infections, that did not bother me. He added that for the next few weeks I would have to take one aspirin every day to thin my blood. That would be the only medication I would need after I left the hospital.

The following days were filled with many visitors, nausea, pain, emotional highs and lows...and my first shampoo in twelve days. Usually I wash my short hair every second day, so after that many days it was beyond description. I desperately wanted it washed, but I was too weak to do it myself. Merv volunteered. A nurse took us to a shower room and somehow he managed. We were told that it was all right if the bandages got wet as they needed to be changed anyway. I discovered that I was cut from just below the breast bone diagonally to the left side just above my waist—23 centimeters (nine inches). A new dressing was applied, I put on a fresh nightgown, and Anita blow dried my hair. I looked and felt like a new person. It's amazing how clean hair can lift one's spirits.

Merv visited me several times each day and brought the

kids in the evening. Sometimes Dave drove straight to the hospital from school, before going to his job.

Due to all the days of IV, my veins stopped cooperating; eventually the only vein they could use was halfway between my wrist and elbow. Only one nurse, who had the nickname Vampire, could find that vein! After the IV was discontinued I was given oral antibiotics instead. My stomach did not tolerate the new medication, so the nausea returned. When I vomit I am very noisy and gag violently. I thought the incision would pop open. I never had to call a nurse. They could always hear me wherever they were and would come running. I would hold my side and lean on the vanity with my hand cushioning the incision. Then I would rest my head on the ledge just above the sink and pray that I would still have a closed wound when the retching had ceased. After a few of those incidents, it was decided to discontinue the oral antibiotics.

My sister sent me a card and letter with jokes every day for a week. As I was getting better each day, those cards were wonderful medicine.

During my stay at the hospital, Dave had the use of my car. One evening while he was working at his job in a local mall someone stole both license plates. Merv reported it and was given some documents to complete. Because it was my car, I had to sign them. I discovered that my vision was really messed up from the drugs. I was unable to read the forms, see the line for my signature, or sit up to sign it. With help from the family, I finally wrote my name in the proper spot. We were not pleased with the thief's timing!

While I was in the hospital, Alf, the husband of my friend Christa, had surgery too. As we were on the same floor, he soon began visiting me. One day I decided that I was well enough to pay him a visit. I grabbed my IV pole and started out, completely unaware that his room was at the far end of the adjoining hall. When I was halfway there I realized that I was too exhausted and sore to go back, so I continued on, hoping that each room I approached would be his.

When I finally found him I dragged myself to the chair and eased myself into it. I certainly was not good company, and I wondered how I would ever get back to my room. We've had many laughs since then about my lively visit with Alf.

My emotions were very unpredictable. Merv's co-workers had sent a large basket filled with all kinds of exotic soaps and lotions. I was delighted as I would never have treated myself like that, but every time I looked at it I cried. That was hard to understand, so I asked Merv to take it home.

The day before I went home, we celebrated Dave's eighteenth birthday in the hospital lounge. Two friends had baked birthday cakes, and we had ice-cream, pop and chips. I didn't eat much, but it was wonderful to be up and around, even though my party attire was a housecoat and slippers.

It was on that day that my head finally cleared. Up until then I had had trouble relating to anything beyond the present time or outside of my hospital room. Spring had brought a heat wave during my last few days in the hospital, and some of my visitors were wearing shorts. That made absolutely no sense, even though I could look out of my window and see the beautiful weather.

Our church is only about two kilometers from the hospital, but on Sunday morning, when I knew that my family and friends would be there, I had no idea where the church was in relation to where I was. It was such a relief to awaken on May 18 and be able to process all those things again.

The next day, two and a half weeks after arriving at the hospital, I was discharged.

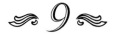

Our friend Helga volunteered to take me home in the morning. That way Merv could go to work for part of the day and be home with me all afternoon. I had promised the ICU nurses that I would say good-bye to them before I left for home. They wanted to see me when I looked like a person again! I went up to the fourth floor to do that. They were astounded that I had healed so fast and that I was walking almost upright, instead of leaning over to the side of my incision. They were obviously very happy for me and joked about how much better I looked now than when they had cared for me.

The ride home was delightful and driving up the long lane was unforgettable. When I had left, winter had barely gone and the leaves were just beginning to show. Now the trees were in full bloom and the lawn and fields were a brilliant green. Home looked so good! I remembered that when Merv and I had driven out, I had wondered if I'd ever drive in that lane again. I went into the house and it seemed to be filled with bouquets, plants and gifts. It was a lovely homecoming.

Just as Helga left, one of Merv's co-workers arrived with a big bouquet and a beautiful musical figurine. I was very thankful for all the kindness that had been shown to me and the family.

Then I went to bed. Our bedroom looked lovely. Merv had cleaned it up and had the window open wide. He had set a fan in the corner, which was circulating the fragrant spring air into every part of the room. As I lay there, I was amazed by the music of the birds. They had arrived while I was gone. It sounded as if I was under a giant canopy filled with the singing of dozens of birds. Many were in the big spreading maple just outside the bedroom window, so the sound was magnificent. As I listened I realized that in amongst all those joyful notes, there were the distant sorrowful strains of the mourning doves which were nesting in the bush. That seemed to complete the picture. Yes, it was good to be home. The cancer was gone, life would go on, but I had come through a very rough experience. Even now when I hear the mourning of doves, I am overwhelmed with feelings of both rejoicing and grieving as I remember that day.

Merv soon arrived home and as he sat by my bed, we thanked God that He had spared me. That evening the next retreatants arrived and I vomited many times during the night. I was sure all twenty of them would hear me. The next day I sat in the sun and breathed in the wonderful spring air.

In the days that followed, Merv and the kids were very good to me, pampering me by doing all the work. That was good because I had absolutely no energy or desire to do anything but sit in our rocking chair. The meals were quite easy for them because our freezer had many casseroles from our church family. It was then that I realized that all the food I had prepared for the family before I was hospitalized was also in the freezer! I had prepared lots of food for them. I hadn't said much to Merv about it because he would have told me not to work so hard. I did not tell Anita, because at that time we had not told the kids of my hospital stay. Well, you guessed it—I had completely forgotten to mention the stockpile of food. Merv had told me that Anita had become the cook, and I assumed that meant thawing and warming the food I had prepared. On the first Sunday, someone at church asked Anita how they were getting along food-wise. She said that she was the cook, but was having trouble trying to figure out what to make. Naturally, the word spread and the casseroles began to arrive—so many that most had to be frozen. So there I was at home, and we had about three weeks worth of prepared food in our freezer! Thank you, Lord, for faithful friends.

❧❧

One evening, about three weeks after I came home, I accidentally bumped my wrist. It hurt much more than it should have. I checked it and there, in a vein, was a small lump which was very tender. We had visitors. Since the woman was nurse, I showed it to her. I thought it was a blood clot and she agreed that it looked like one. Now what!? Blood clots scared me, so I phoned the hospital and was told to come immediately to emergency. Merv and I just looked at each other and shook our heads in disbelief. As we drove up to the hospital, I realized just how much I hated going back.

The doctor saw me very quickly and had good news for us. It was a blood clot, but because it was in one of the veins that had collapsed, it couldn't go anywhere. He told us it would eventually disappear. He assured us that this was quite common after prolonged use of an IV. We went back home feeling very relieved and thankful.

✺ 10 ✺

My nights during that time were very difficult. Pain in my lower back was increasing, and the only relief I could get was to take a hot shower about twice a night. I thought that it was caused by my surgery. After two weeks I phoned the urologist to find out how long the pain would last. He said that I should not be having any pain associated with the surgery. A visit to my chiropractor the next day solved the problem. Apparently back problems are very common after a person has been lifted on and off stretchers and operating tables. I could have saved myself a lot of pain had I not assumed it was a result of my surgery.

Soon after this, I developed a very severe infection in my mouth. It was so swollen I could barely open it. My doctor prescribed antibiotics and suggested that I see my dentist. The dentist told me to come back when I could open my mouth. The infection finally left after the second round of antibiotics. I knew then what the hematologist meant about the increased susceptibility to infections. During that time, my brother and his wife visited with us for a few days. Even though I had to eat and talk through clenched teeth, we had a great time.

⁓⁓

The next few weeks were very different for me. I had gone for walks with my neighbor Nancy almost every day before all this happened. Sometimes we had walked three kilometers, but now I could barely walk to the end of our walkway. Eventually I could get to the end of the lawn and back. Then one morning I phoned Nancy and asked her to come over because I thought I was ready to go for a real walk. Our lane was long and Nancy's lane was just up the road a bit. I was hoping I could walk there and back. But when we were halfway out our lane I knew that if I didn't turn back, Nancy would have to carry me! I always tried very hard to walk upright and had asked my family and Nancy to remind me when I was leaning toward the side of my incision. I was leaning very badly when I reached the house that day.

After several weeks of sitting in the rocking chair all day, I became alarmed. I had always been very active and had enjoyed working (David thought I was crazy), but there I sat with absolutely no ambition. I began to wonder if I would ever have any desire to do anything. I know now from subsequent surgeries that this is how my body reacts to the anesthesia.

At last I woke up one morning feeling ambitious. I had lots of energy and wanted to do some work. I was delighted! Merv was going to do the laundry that evening, but since hanging clothes in the beautiful summer air was one of my favorite jobs, I decided to surprise him. I had a ball! The sky was blue and the clouds were huge and fluffy. The birds were singing and the warm breeze kept away the mosquitoes. Best of all, I was working! I felt like a prisoner let out of a jail cell and I praised the Lord as I went about my tasks. Did I overdo it? Yes, indeed! I sat in my rocking chair for another week. I suppose God knows me well enough that if I would feel ambitious right after surgery, my body would never get the rest it needs.

Eventually, I was given the Pneumovax vaccination and had no more infections. My digestive system took a long time to get back to normal. The vomiting continued until I spent a whole day eating nothing except buttermilk and Astro yogurt which has live culture in it. I was aware that drugs can kill the essential bacteria in the digestive tract, and I knew that those two foods would help them flourish. It worked and I was able to eat regular food again. (McDonald's, get that Egg McMuffin ready!)

One afternoon we visited a woman from our church who was in the last stage of fighting cancer. Bea asked me how I felt about having the disease. I told her that I thought it was just the beginning, as I was facing many tests. Her answer was one that I've remembered often: "Eleanor, it never ends, but you learn to live with it." In late summer I attended her funeral. As I looked at the closed casket at the front of our church I realized once again how close I had come to being there.

11

On June 10, my father, who had fully recovered from his bladder surgery in February, celebrated his 80th birthday. I was disappointed that we missed the family festivities, but I was not strong enough to endure the five-hour trip.

Later in the summer we spent a week at Alf and Christa's cottage which was close enough to Ottawa that I could get to my doctor or the hospital if the need arose. I was almost feeling back to normal and we had a good holiday.

On Thanksgiving weekend we traveled to Pennsylvania to visit friends who had started a Christian community. We always enjoyed our time with them, and since I was feeling fine we had a wonderful trip.

On the second day we went into the city of Williamsport, and Merv did what he always does when he sees a book store. He went in. I went with him, and casually walked the aisles. I spied a large book dealing with cancer. I had read a lot of literature on the subject and had discovered that there was not much written about kidney cancer because it is not very common. Several weeks earlier I had decided that I would stop reading about cancer because I felt I knew all I needed to know. Furthermore, it was irrelevant now that I was well. But my curiosity took over. As I reached for the book I had the feeling that I should not read it. In spite of that I quickly found renal cell cancer in the index. I was delighted. Most books did not even mention it, but this one had enough information to have it listed in the index! As my eyes skimmed the pages, I felt like a child about to get caught with his hand in the cookie jar. Then I saw it. Three-quarters of kidney cancer patients die within the first year. By the end of the fifth year, only a few are alive.

For the first time I felt despair descending on me like a dark cloud. Oh yes, it went on to say that recently immunotherapies had been tried and the results were very encouraging, with more patients surviving. I was well aware that the embolization of my kidney was one of those therapies, but that last bit of information did absolutely nothing to dispel the gloom that was engulfing my whole being. I closed the book, returned it to the shelf and waited in a daze for Merv.

When we were back in the car he realized that something was wrong, so I told him. Somehow he could not understand why I was so upset. That did not surprise me because I couldn't understand it either. It was frightening. All the peace and confidence I had experienced was gone.

I tried to be sociable at the supper table that night, but the dark cloud of despair continued to hang heavily around me.

Before going to bed, the adults of the community household gathered to have a time of Vespers. This included some sharing and praying. I knew I needed help to fight the hopelessness which I felt, so I told them and they prayed. I would like to say that the gloom immediately lifted, but it did not. I was awake far into the night. I prayed and tried to make sense of what had happened. I probably should not have looked into the book, because I really did not need to know any more. Furthermore, when I reached for the book, I had felt a check in my spirit, but I went ahead and read it anyway.

The gloom finally lifted the next day, but looking back, I am thankful that I experienced that dark despair. I can now better empathize with others who encounter those same feelings of hopelessness.

We had a lovely trip back home, and the following months were very busy and rewarding. I enjoyed my time at the retreat house. I was able to share my experiences to encourage others who were also walking in the Valley of the Shadow of Cancer.

❧ 12 ❧

As usual, fall was a magnificent season. The maple bush blazed with a brilliant yellow, and the blue jays began their autumn screaming. Eventually the leaves dropped and the first snows of winter began to gently cover the fields.

In the midst of the retreats we began to make plans for Christmas. I had decided that besides having a large Christmas tree in the retreat lounge, we should have our own tree in our private living room. So one afternoon in early

December I walked the bush and found the perfect little tree. It was only about four feet tall, but it fit beautifully into my big earthenware jug and seemed to be made just for that corner. I quickly decorated it so I could surprise Anita when she came home from school. When she arrived, she was very upset because she had just learned that the mother of one of the girls on her school bus had died of cancer. I was thankful we did not find out until much later that her death was due to kidney cancer. When Anita finished telling me about this, I showed her the little tree. We rejoiced together and continued making our plans for the holiday season.

❧❧

Christmas 1989 was very enjoyable. We traveled to be with the extended family and best of all, seven months after the surgery, I was feeling healthy. My dad remained well, so our family celebrations were joyous.

After the holiday season the retreats resumed and I continued to have my check-ups every three months. These appointments were very easy. I would have a chest x-ray the previous week, so when I'd go to the urologist, he would report that the x-ray was okay and would go on to ask about bone aches and persistent coughing. By God's grace I was always able to reply in the negative. We were very encouraged. There is no chemotherapy for this type of cancer, and since it had not spread to any other organs, I did not need cobalt treatments. Accordingly, I never had to go to the Cancer Clinic.

Since I have a good sense humor, and enjoy a joke on myself, my next chest x-ray at the hospital provided me with a few chuckles. I owned an ugly old Pontiac Phoenix car which we had bought only because the price was right. It had a rust-colored exterior and a red interior. I couldn't imagine anyone buying a new car with that color combination. After the x-ray I went into the parking lot and discovered that my key would not open the car door. As this had never happened before, I pushed, pulled and twisted the key to no avail. I tried the door on the passenger side but with the same result. Standing there feeling stupid, I rechecked that I had the right key. I did. Next I tried the back doors—maybe I had forgotten to lock one. To my delight the rear passenger door was unlocked. I crawled across the back seat and reached forward to unlock the door on the driver's side. As I got out of the car and walked around to the front, a man who had been watching this performance, asked if I needed some help. I thanked him and told him that everything was okay. I put the key into the ignition, but before starting up, I reached over to the passenger seat to get my sunglasses. I saw books on the seat instead of my glasses. For an instant I wondered why I had put books on top of my glasses; then I realized that the books were not mine. What were someone else's books doing in my car? As I inspected the car more closely, I noticed that the stuff on the back window was not mine either! I had gotten into someone else's ugly rust and red Phoenix. I grabbed my keys and with a red face (almost the color of the seats) I quickly vacated the car. I was glad that no one was around, not even the man who had offered his help. I looked around and saw my car one row down from where I was. I have always wondered how far I would have gone before realizing my mistake, if the keys would have started the car.

We had a good laugh when I told my family about my adventure. We had learned by this time that laughter is wonderful therapy in the Valley of the Shadow of Cancer. As Anita always says, "Get those endorphins flowing, Mom."

✎ *13* ✎

*T*he 1990 maple syrup time was delightful. I enjoyed it to the fullest because my health was excellent. We rejoiced that a year had passed since we first entered the Valley.

Since we did not have much of a holiday the previous summer because of my surgery, we made plans to take Anita and her friend Annette with us to Prince Edward Island.

We had a wonderful time on the island, but Merv and I soon realized that the girls would have seen more of the scenery had we taken them to the "Anne of Green Gables" tourist spots later in the week instead of on the first day. They both found L. M. Montgomery books which they had not read, so a lot of their time was spent reading. I must admit that I too almost got hooked with *The Story Girl* and *The Yellow Road*. We had rented a small cabin on a farm, and between sightseeing and relaxing it was a great holiday.

One night near the end of our stay, I awoke and as I turned my head in the darkness to check the time, I noticed what seemed to be rings of light flashing before my eyes. As I lay there I saw them every time I moved my head. When I discovered that they were visible with my eyes open or closed, I became very frightened. I knew that kidney cancer is notorious for traveling to the brain, and I also was aware that visual disturbances are sometimes the first signs of a tumor. After praying, I decided that I would not tell anyone until we were back home. By God's grace I fell asleep.

The next morning the sun was shining into our bedroom. I quickly moved my head. The flashing rings were not visible. I discovered that night that I could only see them in the dark.

We spent our last day in Charlottetown, and in the evening we went to see the musical performance of *Anne of Green Gables*. It was fabulous and any thoughts of a possible brain tumor were far away.

The trip home was tense as it was the time of the uprising at the Oka Reserve. The aboriginal peoples were threatening to close roads and bomb bridges, and our route took us very close to that area. I prayed a lot for our safety and my health.

David had not gone with us. He needed to stay at his job to make money for his first year of university. He was a collector and a skateboarder, so he had parts of skateboards and other "treasures" scattered in the basement. We would be arriving home just before school started so I had kidded him that I wouldn't let him move out until he had cleaned up his mess in the basement. (We either had to buy a third car or have him live in town. We chose the latter.)

When we arrived home it was evening. All Dave's furniture was in the lobby. A note on the kitchen table welcomed us back and told us that he and his friend Trevor would be moving the next day. This was my first child leaving home and I was proud of myself—I didn't feel sorry that he was going. Instead I felt very happy and excited for him. My reaction surprised me because, as a stay-at-home mom, I doted on and overprotected my kids. The next day I happened to go into the basement and I was shocked. Dave had cleaned up his mess; in fact it was all gone. He had not left one bit of his stuff behind. I fought back the tears because it looked as though he had never existed. I had asked him to clean up, but I guess I still wanted some remnants of his childhood to be visible. I called Anita down, said nothing, and watched her reaction. She was just about to ask what I wanted when she looked at Dave's part of the basement and her mouth dropped. She stood there and said, "Oh Mom." It was down there that this mother and daughter realized that their family of four would now be a family of three for most of the time. We were quiet as we climbed the stairs. I was suddenly very glad that he was moving only to Ottawa.

We helped Dave and his friend move, and the fall retreats began.

≈ 14 ≈

It was exciting to get back into the routine of retreats, but

I still had to get those flashing rings checked out. I started by going to my chiropractor. I expressed my concerns about a brain tumor. He thought it was a neck problem since it only happened when I moved my head while lying down. If it was caused by a tumor, the position of my head and neck probably would not influence it. He adjusted my spine and neck, but the flashing rings continued to appear. After a few more appointments he suggested that I should see a neurologist. That was put on hold because I had an optometrist's appointment. When I told the optometrist about my cancer, as well as the visual disturbances, he became very serious and spent a long time doing tests and examining my eyes more thoroughly than ever before. He didn't find anything unusual. He gave me a new prescription and advised me to see a neurologist. I knew that I couldn't delay any longer, but I had a problem. I had not told Merv about the flashing rings. I hadn't wanted to spoil our holidays by telling him then, and an appointment with the chiropractor was not unusual. Now I had to explain my upcoming visit to the neurologist.

That evening when Merv and I were waiting in the car for Anita's Youth Group to end, I told him. His reaction was not what I had expected. He was very angry at me for not telling him. I really had thought it was a neck problem which could be corrected by a few chiropractic adjustments, so it would serve no purpose for Merv to know. I was only trying to protect him from worrying, but he felt rejected, angry and left out.

This is something those in the Valley need to deal with, because similar situations happen so frequently. As the patient, I want to shield my loved ones from some of the emotional pain, but as the spouse, Merv wants to share the pain and feels rejected when I choose to carry it by myself. This is one aspect of living with cancer that we still have difficulty sorting out. Our ride home that evening was very quiet and tense.

↝∘↜

After several weeks the neurology appointment became a reality rather than a monster looming in the distance. The neurologist was very pleasant. He had Merv and me laughing many times as he proceeded with the examination. He finally said that he could find no problems; I did not have a brain tumor, but he would arrange an appointment with a retinal specialist and a booking for a CAT scan of the brain. No tumor and yet a CAT scan? Why? He said it would be more for my reassurance than anything else. I would have felt more at ease leaving his office if he had not mentioned the scan.

The CAT scan was scheduled for early January '91. That Christmas we traveled to celebrate the season with family. I remember standing in my parents' home, staring out into the darkness. Everyone else had gone to bed, so I was alone. I thought of my two other minor concerns. Sometimes I felt a very small twinge of pain in my lungs. I probably would not have noticed it had I not been aware that kidney cancer spreads to the lungs. Also, since our trip, my back was occasionally very sore. Again this was a problem only because I knew that this type of cancer spreads to the bones, especially the spine. I thought now of the many times the urologist had asked if I had any bone aches. I wondered if I would be alive next Christmas.

≈ 15 ≈

The retreats resumed shortly after the holidays, and the activities helped keep my mind off the upcoming CAT scan. Several of our friends were praying for us and I had peace.

During this waiting period I started having rectal bleeding. I was devastated. What else could possibly happen? I made an appointment with the rectal surgeon who had repaired my hemorrhoids several years earlier. He started the examination by asking me about my health in general. When I told him about my bout with cancer, he immediately began to feel around my collar bone. A cold chill swept over me as I realized he was searching for swollen lymph glands—a sign that the disease has spread. He then got down to the business at hand! I have yet to experience anything more embarrassing and humiliating than a rectal examination. He quickly found the source of the bleeding. I had a tiny rip in the bowel, probably caused by a hard piece of Christmas nut as it traveled through my body. When he asked if I had taken any drugs recently, I told him that I had been taking some aspirin for a headache. That, of course, had thinned my blood, making the bleeding more profuse. Another crisis was over, but in a few days I would be facing the scan.

Merv took me to the hospital for the scan, and as I waited for my name to be called, I had mixed emotions. The peace that passes understanding was present, but so was the fear of the unknown.

After a rather long wait I was taken into the CAT scan room, and was assured that the procedure would not hurt. A needle was inserted into the back of my hand and through it the dye, a colorless liquid, entered my body. The scan was uneventful and I was soon put into a tiny room by myself. I began to shake uncontrollably. That reminded me of the shakes I had experienced after giving birth. Since that had been caused by the epidural drugs, I assumed that I was reacting to the dye. I felt very lonely and abandoned, so I prayed. A nurse finally came and said that I could go home. She told me I would have the results in about two weeks.

The next week I went to the retinal specialist who did all sorts of strange tests on my eyes. I began to wonder if I would ever be able to see properly again. When he was finished he informed me that I had Moore's Lightning Streaks. He provided an explanation of the cause, of which I understood absolutely nothing, except that it was no problem whatsoever. That news made it easier to wait for the scan results, since we knew for sure that the cause of my visual problems was not a brain tumor. Even so, I was very relieved when I received the phone call reporting that the CAT scan showed no abnormality. Thank you, Lord. Things were back to normal again; even the discomfort in my lungs and back had completely disappeared.

❧❧

The maple syrup season arrived again, and we thanked God that in spite of some crises I was now in good health, ready for the extra work and fun this time of year brought with it.

I had my yearly physical and all was well. I made an appointment for my yearly mammogram. Three days before I went, I discovered a lump in my left breast. I had developed many breast lumps and cysts in the past, and I always went to the doctor immediately. Most could be aspirated, proving that they were cysts, therefore not malignant. The one which had been surgically removed was benign. Since I was having a mammogram in three days, I decided to wait and see if this new lump would show up. The mammogram results showed no malignant tumors, so my new lump was no problem, right?

On May 4, 1991, Merv came home with a bouquet to celebrate two years of good health. God had been very good to us and I vowed to myself that I would never worry about my health again.

❧❧

After retreats stopped for the summer, I did a lot of weeding in our large garden. This involved prolonged periods of bending which made my left side (the site of my kidney surgery) very uncomfortable. By fall when the retreats resumed, I realized that something was very wrong in that side, just under my incision. It felt as though some foreign object, about the size of a lemon, was in there. Even though I couldn't feel it with my hand, it was very uncomfortable when I bent over or wore a tight belt. I could feel it with every step I took. I finally phoned the urologist, and he

-49-

suggested that I have an ultrasound. I cringed at the thought of more tests, but I had to find out what was causing this new problem.

I had not been told to fast, and the little box on the back of the requisition which indicates the need for a fast was not checked. So on the morning of the ultrasound I had a large breakfast. That was a mistake. The technician asked why I hadn't fasted. I told her, and she said that it was no use to continue because of all the food in my stomach. What a disappointment. Another appointment was set up, and that time I fasted longer than was necessary. I did not worry about the results. I remembered all the other false alarms and tried to convince myself that this would be one too.

❧❧

A week later I was peeling apples with three friends from church when the phone rang. We were making applesauce to be used at retreats, and as usual, we were having a good time. I answered the phone. It was the urologist. He informed me that he was booking an abdominal CAT scan because the ultrasound did not show a clear picture of my left side. He mentioned something about the bowel and not being able to see behind it, but my heart was beating so hard and my head was spinning so fast that I didn't ask him to explain it better. My understanding was that there was a bowel problem, and I assumed that the CAT scan would show whether or not it was malignant. I hung up and slowly walked to the kitchen. Again I was devastated and knew that I would need a lot of prayer. I told my friends at the table and they immediately put down their knives and apples and we prayed. When I told Merv that night, we tried to be strong for each other, but it was hard not to show our disappointment. Even though I knew God was in control and that He would give me peace, I began to wonder what He was doing.

The CAT scan was in the evening several weeks later, and as we walked down the quiet hospital hall I felt numb. As I looked at Merv's ashen face, I said, choking back my tears,

"Will it never end?" I thought back to Bea's words to me.

I was given a thick white liquid to drink. Then I was taken into the room. The stretcher I was on was positioned in the machine. The instructions, "Hold your breath...Breathe...," continued throughout the whole procedure. I felt at peace when we left the hospital, but the next week was tense.

By Thursday, every time the phone rang my blood pressure shot up and my heart felt as if it was going to leap right out of my ribcage. By the time I had walked down the hall to the phone my throat was completely dry. I was disappointed at my reaction. Since I believed that my health was in God's hands, I had peace, but the phone freaked me out. Because the phone at a retreat house rings frequently, I ran to the phone many times, only to have a pastor on the other end wanting to make a booking. By Friday I was totally uptight. Again I had peace about what might happen, but I dreaded the phone call. Finally the urologist called and told me that the scan was normal. He explained that when my kidney, spleen and tumor were removed two and a half years earlier, the space that was created was taken over by my bowel. This is quite normal, but in my case the bowel had several loops in it which caused my discomfort. There definitely was no cancer. I was very ashamed that I had been so upset and asked God to forgive me for my lack of faith. I realized that, "Do not fret, it leads only to evil"(Ps. 37:8b), was a verse that still needed some work for me. Another crisis had passed, but I felt as though I had been in the Valley for a long, long time.

∽ 16 ∾

*F*all '91 came with its usual display of glory. The maple bush was brilliant, and I thanked God daily for the privilege of being alive to enjoy it. Retreatants came and went, and any thoughts of cancer were quickly dismissed.

In my morning devotions I had started the November-December '91 *Every Day With Jesus* booklet. The topic was "Riding the Winds of Adversity." I was very thankful that my life at present had no adversity, but the study was very meaningful. All the scripture verses were those that had sustained me during my hard times. In mid-November I had my regular appointment with the urologist. I awoke that morning feeling great because I already had the results of the CAT scan and I had no other problems to discuss with him.

As I lay there in the semi-darkness, I realized that the only concern left was that lump in my breast. It had not shown up on the mammogram, but that was seven months ago, so maybe I should have it checked. It would be good to hear the doctor tell me that if it didn't show up on the mammogram it was okay. I phoned his office and was told to come after my appointment with the urologist.

The urologist had the results of my chest x-ray taken the previous week, and it was clear. My heart sang as I left his office. In a few minutes I would have the lump checked and I would have a clean bill of health.

When I told the doctor that I had not come to him sooner because the lump had not shown up on the mammogram, he said I should have come. Apparently one should not depend on that procedure in making a decision about a breast lump. I was shocked. What were mammograms for if they weren't accurate in diagnosing lumps? He was unable to aspirate the lump. It was not a cyst. That was not very encouraging. He suggested that even though he did not think that it was malignant, he wanted a second opinion. He would book an appointment with a surgeon. I cannot find any words to describe my disappointment. That night I had more news for Merv.

Shortly before this, a family had moved in with us, and I

had decided to go back into teaching as a supply teacher. I was teaching the morning of my appointment with the surgeon, so I left the school and went straight to the medical building where I met Merv. Overall, I felt little anxiety. The mammogram had been clear, my doctor thought it was benign, so I was there to have that confirmed because of my age and medical history. When I was called into the surgeon's office I asked Merv to come in with me. The doctor asked when I had discovered the lump, and I stressed that with every other lump I had always gone to the doctor the next day, but because of the mammogram, I had assumed that this one was okay. He said the same as the other doctor—mammograms should not be relied on to diagnose lumps. I felt betrayed. No one had ever told me that. I knew that breast x-rays were not always accurate in finding tiny lumps, but I thought they were very accurate with larger ones that could be felt. I have since asked many of my friends, including several nurses, and they also had believed the same myth.

I went into the examining room and stripped from the waist up. Before he even examined me he said that he never leaves a lump in the breast of a woman my age, therefore this one would have to be surgically removed. He examined my breasts very carefully and left. I dressed, went back into his office and sat beside Merv. The surgeon told us the procedure. I would have a general anesthesia. Then he would remove the lump and some of the surrounding tissue. This would be sent to the lab for an immediate diagnosis. If it was benign I could go home the same evening. If it was malignant, he would continue the surgery by removing several lymph nodes from my armpit and inserting a drainage tube. I would be in the hospital for three days. I couldn't believe what I was hearing. When he was finished explaining, I asked him if there was anything about the lump that made him think it was malignant and he said there wasn't.

The surgery was scheduled for the next week and I had total peace for most of the time. The fact that he had said that I needed surgery before examining me was reassuring. I was told that he was an excellent doctor, so he was just being very careful.

The day before the surgery I received a call from the hospital to remind me to fast and to arrive well ahead of the surgery time. The secretary then asked if our insurance allowed for a ward or a semi-private room. I said that I would probably be going home the same day. She replied, "But you are booked in for three days." I managed to say that that didn't sound good and she agreed. I hung up the phone and walked around in a state of severe disappointment and bewilderment. Merv comforted me by saying that the doctor probably always booked his patients in so that in case of a problem there would be a bed available. It did not necessarily mean I would be staying.

The next morning I was feeling fine. Many people were praying for us and I felt calm. We went to the hospital and after I disrobed I waited with Merv. It seemed like a dream, but I was very confident that this was a false alarm. Finally I was wheeled into the OR and went to sleep saying the Twenty-third Psalm.

After what seemed like a few minutes I awoke in the recovery room. I drifted in and out of sleep and finally woke up enough to check if there was a drainage tube protruding from my arm pit. The entire left side of my chest and up into my arm pit was bandaged. Since the lump had been in the upper left quadrant of my breast it did not surprise me that the dressing would extend that high. I felt very carefully for a tube and found none. I was relieved; no drain meant no cancer. I dozed off with a prayer of gratitude in my heart. The next time I awoke, my arm bumped against something hard just above my breast bone. I grabbed at the covers and my gown and pulled them away from my body to see what the hard object was. The unbelievable was happening. I saw a small plastic reservoir into which was draining a light pink fluid. There was a drain! I had breast cancer!

Just then an attendant came and wheeled me to my room where Merv was waiting. I said, "It is," and he replied, "I know." There are times when silence says more than words. We were both hurting very badly. The surgeon told us that it was a small tumor and he had been able to remove all of it. In about a week we would have the lab report of the six lymph nodes he had removed. I asked why he had done a lumpectomy instead of a mastectomy, and he assured me that a lumpectomy plus radiation treatments was just as effective. Merv phoned our pastor and started the prayer chain on my behalf. What a blessing to have dozens of friends praying.

I knew that at six o'clock that evening the outdoor Christmas lights at the hospital were to be turned on for the first time. I really didn't care.

After supper I phoned my parents, stressing that it was a little lump and that I'd be home in three days. Having had breast cancer herself, my mother was very concerned, but we were encouraged that she was a survivor. I phoned a sister-in-law, and after her shock she promised to have her prayer group intercede for me also. She was very encouraging, and we managed to laugh and cry together. Merv, Dave and Anita came to see me that night, and once again I tried to be one hundred per cent positive for the kids. I found out later from my mother that she had phoned that evening and had asked Anita what she thought about her mother having cancer again. Her answer was typical of Anita: "She'll be okay, Grandma. Jesus is with her."

Since this had not been major surgery, I felt great the next day and walked the halls a lot. The surgeon was surprised to see me doing so well. What discouraged me the most was that I had another kind of cancer. I expressed that concern to my doctor and the nurses, and they all said the same thing. This was much better than having a return of the kidney cancer. *That* would be disastrous!

◈

That afternoon I had a very special experience. I don't know if I was fully awake or asleep. I saw a page of a calendar. Instead of the lines forming squares to mark each day, there were walls surrounding each day creating boxes. With that, I heard the words, "You must not go out of your box for today." I believed it was a message from the Lord and it obviously meant that I should live one day at a time and have no worries about the future (Matt. 6:34). I couldn't understand why He would show me this, since I had spent very little time worrying. Yes, there were many tense times, but with prayer, peace always returned. He obviously knew more about what lay in the future than I did.

The next day I went home. The *Every Day With Jesus* devotions continued to be a source of strength, especially now that I was going through adversity. One idea really got my attention. It said that in adversity one should not ask why, but rather ask God how He can use you in the situation. I did that and saw it as an opportunity to tell others of His love.

The day after I returned home there was a retreat for which we were providing the food. Several women came, and I sat in the kitchen giving instructions since I had planned the menu and had begun preparations before my surgery. We did a lot of laughing and joking in spite of the fact that once again I was walking in the Valley of the Shadow of Cancer.

≈ *17* ≈

*O*n Monday morning, five days after my surgery, Merv went to the doctor and this became one of the most devastating days of my life. He had been working far too much and while I saw it, he didn't. He had done more than eighty-eight hours overtime in one month for his job. He also did an incredible amount of work in the upkeep of the retreat property and had eldership duties at church. I had been praying for him as I feared he would suffer from a burnout. I had hoped that having the other family there would give him a break, but there was always much more that had to be done. My breast cancer seemed to be the last straw. He phoned at lunch time to tell me that the doctor had recommended he be off work for three months. This was a great blow. Merv had always been the strong one for me, and now he was in the midst of a burnout.

I had not received the lab report on my lymph nodes, so I did not know my prognosis. If the nodes were free of cancer I would probably have cobalt treatments, but if malignant cells were found, chemotherapy would be advised.

I know that God promises never to send more than we can handle, but that day came very close to going beyond that point. I spent most of the afternoon walking the trails in the bush crying out to God in utter desperation. I interceded for Merv and couldn't help but wonder how we would cope with a burnout and cancer while running a retreat house. I tried hard to stay in my "box for today."

I phoned all the schools in which I had been supplying, to tell them not to call until further notice because of my cancer surgery. I wondered if I would ever be able to phone them back to inform them that I was available.

Tuesday was Merv's first day home and we tried to adjust to this new situation. I began to realize that our time at that place was probably drawing to a close. Neither of us was in a position to keep up with the hectic pace of living at a very busy retreat house.

The next day we had to do some shopping and decided that going out for lunch might help to relieve the despair and tension we both felt. Merv had gone out to warm up the car, and just as I was going out the door to join him I heard the phone ring. I rushed in and received the good news that the lymph nodes were clean. The cancer had not spread! I laughed and cried, phoned my parents, and then ran out to the car to tell Merv. Needless to say, we had a wonderful lunch.

On Thursday, after the stitches were removed, I went to a Cursillo weekend (a time apart for studying the deeper Christian life) that I had registered for many weeks earlier. I usually have a very good sense of humor, but that evening as I sat in my small group of women, all of whom were strangers, nothing was humorous. My breast hurt from having the stitches removed, and I was very concerned about Merv.

Finally, I explained to the women why I was being so unsociable. The woman beside me leaned over, put her hand on my shoulder and said, "You'll be okay. I had cancer and Jesus healed me too." It seemed as though an angel had spoken those words. She later shared with me that she had had uterine cancer and that after much prayer and a specialized diet combined with drugs, she was healed. (Since then she has had two healthy babies.) I hung on to her words and hoped that the Holy Spirit had prompted her to say them.

I had heard of fighting cancer with diet, vitamins and other immune system boosters, and I knew of a holistic medical doctor who used those methods. I had prayed for wisdom to know whether or not I should make an appointment to see him. Over that weekend I met another woman who had survived cancer by going on a very strict diet and boosting her immune system. I felt that was a confirmation, so shortly after I returned home I phoned that doctor. The fact that he was a medical doctor and a dedicated Christian was very important to me.

❧❧

By now it was mid-December, so we decided that I should write our Christmas letters. After the fifth one telling about my latest battle with cancer, I quit. Only five people received Christmas greetings that year.

I soon learned that I would need five weeks of cobalt treatments starting in early January '92. The thought of driving into the city every morning in an Ottawa winter would have been nerve-racking, but with Merv home, I would have a chauffeur. This was an excellent example of Romans 8:28: "And we know that in all things, God works for the good of those who love Him, who have been called according to His purpose."

The Christmas tree was put up, but I have no recollection of ever sitting by it or enjoying it. Merv's burnout and the upcoming cobalt treatments were taking their toll on us even though we felt God's presence and knew Him to be with us. We had our usual Christmas celebrations with the extended family, and again after the long drive I had a very bad backache. Was it from sitting in the car so long, or had one of the cancers spread to my spine? During our visit, we had the use of our friends' home in Stratford while they were in Winnipeg celebrating Christmas with their family. It was a great blessing for us to have our own space at that particular time.

Right after Christmas we were invited to spend a few days in Pennsylvania with our friends. We had a blessed time. It was so good to get away from all the reminders of the difficulties we were facing. It taught me that an invitation extended to hurting people can be a wonderful ministry. We were very thankful for the care our friends gave us.

On the weekend before the start of my cobalt treatments, Merv and I accepted another invitation from friends at a retreat house in the Finger Lake area in New York state. This was an unforgettable experience. For a change I was on the receiving end at a retreat house, and I enjoyed the prepared meals immensely. We stayed there until the morning of my first appointment in the radiology department at the Cancer Clinic, and our friends prayed with us before we left. My feelings regarding the treatments were quite positive, but I had an uneasiness about the big cobalt machine. I suppose it was fear of the unknown.

❧ *18* ❧

My first visit to the Cancer Clinic was uneventful. I saw many people in the waiting room. Some were wearing green robes and others were dressed in street clothes. It was obvious that the robed ones were the patients and the others were loved ones who had come to give their support. I was secretly very happy that the green shade of the robes happened to be one of my best colours. I would be needing all the help I could get to avoid looking sickly. I met the radiation oncologist and all the information was taken. My breast was marked with blue marker. I was advised to wear cotton bras and blouses because the treatments that would start the next day would cause a "sunburn." Cotton is the most comfortable material.

During the next five weeks I was not to wash my left breast or armpit with soap, in fact, the less water the better. Deodorants and antiperspirants were forbidden, as was showering. No showers for five weeks seemed inconceivable. By the second week of no soap, little water and no deodorant, I kidded Merv that he should always sit upwind from me. For the first time in my life I had body odor. I joked with the radiation technicians about it and sometimes said, "Here comes the armpit!" as I walked into the treatment room. They laughed and assured me that all their breast cancer patients were very aware of their armpits during the treatments.

In each treatment the radiation was beamed on each side of my breast for approximately one minute. I lay on a flat table with my breast clamped between two pieces of plastic.

This was quite uncomfortable and I felt very confined, but it didn't last long. During the treatment the technicians left the room, but they always reminded me that they could see and hear me if I called to them. That was comforting. I always said the Twenty-third Psalm silently during the first half and the Lord's Prayer during the second.

The first two weeks went very well, as I had absolutely no discomfort. Merv and I would often leave home early so we would have time for coffee and a muffin in the hospital cafeteria. Sometimes we treated ourselves to a whole breakfast. I was so thankful that Merv was able to be with me.

During the third week I found a lump in my other breast, and even though it was not my day to see the oncologist, I asked to see him. He was very reassuring and we both were relieved when he was able to aspirate the new lump. I shared with him how awful I felt that seven months had been lost because I had depended on the mammogram. This was especially hard for me to accept because the mistake was made on the only one that was malignant. All my other lumps had been checked out immediately. I felt there was no justice in that. The oncologist cautioned me to stop thinking about those seven months. Breast cancer takes from seven to nine years to develop fully, so he felt that the lost time would not have made much difference, especially since it had not spread to the lymph system. I felt at ease as I left his office.

Because I have my dad's dark complexion, my skin tans easily, so the rest of the treatment time was relatively easy for me. Yes, I did get a "sunburn," and an open sore developed in my armpit, but with the help of cortisone cream and prayer, I healed very quickly.

My five weeks of treatments ended the day before Anita's seventeenth birthday. It was a great celebration. I was very thankful to be alive for the occasion, and Merv and I were relieved that our early morning trips to Ottawa were finished.

I experienced the most discomfort the week after the treatments ended, but finally the big day arrived—my first shower! How could something so ordinary give me such pleasure? I was not concerned about saving water that day.

A week later I visited all the schools and asked them to put me back on their lists. Merv took a picture of me standing beside my car on the first day I went back teaching. My smile says it all. I sang praise songs all the way.

My appointment with the holistic physician finally arrived. After going over the questionnaire I had filled out, and asking Merv and me many questions, he concluded that heredity probably was a large factor in my health situation. It appeared that my immune system needed some help, so he prescribed many different vitamins and minerals as well as lots of beta carotene. We talked about the spiritual side of illness as well, and we left his office feeling that we had found a friend who was willing to help.

☙❧

By April '92, Merv was back at work part time, and we began searching for a new home. It seemed clear to us that God was showing us that our time at the retreat house was over. We continued trying to stay in our "box for today," but that was difficult as I had not received a salary at the retreat house, and house prices had gone up considerably since we had sold ours seven years earlier.

About that time, as I turned in bed one morning, I felt what seemed to be a lump on my right shoulder blade. In a panic I felt very carefully, and indeed there was a lump a bit bigger than a marble. It was oblong, smooth, and just under the skin. It caused no bulge, but I could roll it around under my fingers. Since it was only about three inches from my armpit I thought it was a lymph node. That was frightening as it was not on the side where I had had breast cancer. Had it spread? Would it never end?

I went to see a doctor the same day and was assured that it was a lipoma, which is a fatty lump, never malignant and never a problem. I asked if I should keep an eye on it, but was told to forget about it. I was very relieved, because all my thoughts were focused on house hunting. I really had no time to deal with yet another bout with cancer.

After a lot of searching and continuous prayer, we put in an offer on a house. It was very close to Anita's high school, and Merv would have about the same distance to work as he had from the retreat house. It was three blocks from a sandy beach along a bay on the Ottawa River. We asked God to shut the door if this wasn't to be ours, but everything worked out. On June 15th, we moved into our new home. We had been at the retreat house almost seven years so it was different to be by ourselves, working for ourselves instead of for others. The house and property needed a lot of work, so we spent the summer landscaping the badly neglected lot.

During the summer, shortly before my regular checkup at the Cancer Clinic, I found a new lump in my right breast. That meant I had two lumps that needed to be checked. I had decided to also show those doctors the lump on my shoulder to get a second opinion, even though I had been told that it was okay. In mid July, the Cancer Clinic doctors agreed that the lump on my shoulder was a lipoma. They did not find the new lump in my breast, but when I pointed it out to them they panicked and called in another doctor. They tried to aspirate it, but were unable to withdraw any fluid. That was bad news. A needle biopsy was done, and I was told to have a mammogram and see my surgeon as soon as possible. Once again I lay on an examining table in utter disbelief. It seemed like a very bad dream. Somehow I managed to get dressed while crying out to God to strengthen me and help me tell Merv.

Merv's burnout, my disease and our move had emotionally drained both of us. We had hoped that things would improve in our new home. But there we were, barely moved in, facing another crisis. When I got to the waiting room, Merv had gone out to "feed" the parking meter, so while I waited for him I phoned the surgeon's office. His secretary could hear my devastation. She tried to comfort me, but couldn't hide the dismay in her voice. I asked if the doctor was in, and she told me to come immediately. He was one of the few doctors I still trusted, and she sensed how desperately I needed to see him. Merv returned and as we left the clinic I told him the news. As we drove to the doctor's office, guilt overwhelmed me. How could I put my family through this again? Anita's confirmation was in two weeks and we would be having visitors. How could I have surgery? We both prayed silently until we arrived at the medical building.

The surgeon saw me immediately and was very encouraging. He couldn't understand why the Cancer Clinic doctors had been in such a flap. As far as he was concerned it was a fibrous mass—nothing to be concerned about. I was almost afraid to believe him, but I was very relieved. The thought of showing him the lump on my shoulder never crossed my mind.

~⧲∘⧳~

The next week I had my mammogram, and a few days later I got a call from the oncologist at the Cancer Clinic. The results of both the needle biopsy and mammogram were negative. When I told her what the surgeon had said, she said that nothing further would be done. I was to watch it and come back to the Cancer Clinic in a month. She explained that while a mammogram or a needle biopsy are not always accurate on their own, if both are negative and the surgeon agrees, chances are very good that there is no malignancy. That certainly was excellent news as Anita's confirmation was now only a few days away. Again we had not told the kids about this crisis and we thanked God that the prognosis was good. In a month I returned to the Cancer Clinic, and the doctors were totally certain that the lump was benign.

By the time summer turned into fall, most of our landscaping was finished, Merv had returned to a full-time work schedule, and my thoughts turned to indoor decorating and supply teaching. I was feeling very healthy, so without the extra work of the retreat house I was hoping to do a lot of teaching. The decorating would need some extra money. I visited the schools close by and prayed that I would be called to work in spite of a surplus of supply teachers.

Fall was beautiful, but we soon found out that the oak leaves, which had been lovely during the summer, became a nuisance when they finally dropped in late fall. We have about forty oak trees on our lot, and we were literally up to our knees in leaves. Our neighbors, who had learned to cope with this autumn deluge, kidded us every time we were out raking. We finished the task just as the first snow began to fall. This prompted Anita and me to start planning for Christmas. The previous Christmas season was one we wanted to forget. This year would be wonderful in our new home. We loved lighting the fireplace, and as we sat there we planned where we would put our Christmas tree. We all looked forward to Dave coming home for the holidays. Anita and I kept reminding ourselves how much better this Christmas would be.

≈ 19 ≈

*I*ndeed, life *was* going well. Merv was relaxed and very happy in our new home, Dave was succeeding in university, Anita was very happy to be in the same school which was only a five minute drive away, and I was faithfully taking my vitamins and beta carotene and staying in my "box for today." I also began to get teaching jobs which was a pleasure. Once again cancer was in the past.

In late November '92, my regular six month urology appointment indicated that I was fine. In early December, I had my checkup with the surgeon. Since I had no new breast lumps, this was to be a very fast in and out appointment, so I told Merv that he didn't have to come with me. He insisted, so we agreed to meet at the mall and we'd go together from there. That way we would pay parking fees for only one car.

On my way I stopped to get our mail. There were several pieces. One was a rather drab looking postcard with a poem on it. I arrived at the mall before Merv so I looked at the mail. The postcard was from Gloria, a partially disabled friend who had spent many weeks with us over the years while we lived at the retreat house. She wished us a Merry Christmas and invited us to visit her over the holidays. The poem on the front was really a song by Annie Johnson Flint:

He Giveth Me More Grace

He giveth more grace when the burdens grow greater,
He sendeth more strength when the labors increase;
To added affliction He addeth His mercy
To multiplied trials, His multiplied peace.
His love has no limit; His grace has no measure;
His power no boundary known unto men;
For out of His infinite riches in Jesus
He giveth and giveth and giveth again.

As I put it into my purse, I thought that those words would be very comforting if I had been expecting this to be a bad appointment. The postcard was not particularly relevant that day, even though I had experienced those graces in the past. Merv came, and with our spirits high, we drove off to the surgeon's office. After I had once again "stripped from the waist up" I felt chilly, so I wrapped my arms around myself, and my hand touched the lump on my shoulder. Yes, it was still there, but the other doctors had said that it was a lipoma so there was no need to show this doctor. Part of me wanted to get his opinion, but I decided I was getting paranoid. Before I had made the final decision whether or not to tell him about the lump, he walked in with a young doctor. Without thinking, I showed it to him. I could tell immediately by his expression that he did not like it. I told him what the other doctors had said, but he just kept on feeling it. He had the young doctor examine it, and finally I asked if it was a lipoma. He said it was not.

My heart sank. I asked what it was. He said he didn't know, so it had to come out. It had been seven months since I had been told that the lump was a lipoma! Then he checked my breasts, and when I mentioned the lump that he had checked in June, he said he still felt the same about it, but since I was having surgery anyway, he would remove it too. This couldn't be happening! What about my supply teaching? What about our plans for Christmas? He knew I was very upset, so he said that I could continue my teaching as he did not have an opening in the operating room until December 21, which was in the holidays. He thought I probably would be well enough to continue teaching when school reopened in January. Somehow those words had a hollow ring to them because I was facing surgery again. I got dressed, walked into the waiting room, shook my head at Merv, grabbed my coat and almost ran out the door. I was supposed to have told the receptionist to book me for surgery on the 21st, but I just couldn't. I phoned her the next day. Somewhere between the shut door and the elevator, I told Merv about the upcoming surgery four days before Christmas. I began to identify with Job.

As this was a very grey, damp, December day, as dismal as my spirits, Merv thought it would be wise for me to spend some time with a friend in the city before going home. We phoned Michele. She was on her way out, but told me to come anyway. She could go out later. I poured out the whole story, and she grieved too. For many years, we had been meeting regularly with her and her husband and another couple, studying the Christian way of life and praying together. She had walked with us through all the other problems.

While Michele and I were praying, I suddenly remembered the postcard. It was *very relevant* after all. I read it to her, and she immediately said, "Eleanor, that's from the Lord!" It was quite strange that Gloria would have sent it to us, so I phoned to ask her about it without telling her the news I had just received. She said that she thought that the Lord wanted her to send it. She had wanted to write us a note. She had many pretty notecards and postcards, but her attention was always drawn to that rather drab one. She really did not want to send it because it was so plain, but finally she chose it because she felt she should. She was sorry to hear that I was facing surgery again, but we rejoiced that she had been obedient and had sent me the card with those encouraging words on it. Michele laughed and said, "You're in goods hands, Eleanor! Now the Lord even sends you postcards." Then we prayed and she read the words on the postcard in the first person, as if God Himself was saying them. "I give more grace...I send more strength..."

As I left her house the emotional hurting had ceased, and once again I had hope. At least God knew everything that was happening, and I believed with my whole heart that He had used Gloria to send me those words. I had told Merv that I would not tell Anita right away, but he knew I could not hide my disappointment, so we decided to tell her. I prayed on the way home that God would show me the right time and give me the right words. There were times when I was very concerned about the effect my continuing health struggles would have on our kids' faith.

Anita arrived home shortly after I did. She had received

the results of some tests and the marks were all super. Best of all she had no homework for the first time in months. She thought we should phone Merv and meet him in town for supper. When she finished telling me about her day, I told her about mine. Anita was excited about the postcard, said a few angry things about the other doctors, and then commented that we really had to be thankful for the surgeon's caution. Her reaction was excellent, so I phoned Merv and arranged to meet him for supper, even though we had never done that before. Only the Lord can arrange a celebration on the same day as receiving devastating news!

We were expecting company the next evening, so I started to clean the house before it was time to leave to meet Merv. As I was dusting I suddenly remembered the sticker on the back of the postcard. I had noticed when I first saw it, that it had some printing on it. It was probably a scripture, but I had not read it. Somehow, I now felt it was important, and as I walked into the bedroom to get it, I told myself that this was going to be the icing on the cake! And indeed it was. It was Psalm 50:15: "Call upon me in the day of trouble and I will deliver thee and thou shalt glorify me." What joy! Was He really going to deliver me? It was so appropriate because for several months I had been praying special prayers that I would glorify God in my life. This was an answer to my prayers. I showed it to Anita and we rejoiced together.

The next day I began to wonder why Gloria would have chosen that particular sticker since she knew nothing of what I would be facing. In fact, I didn't even know about it when she had sent it. I phoned and put that question to her. She chuckled, saying that I probably wouldn't believe it. She had awakened in the middle of the night with the feeling that she should look for something. She got up and went around the room, realizing how ridiculous that was. How could she find something if she didn't know what she was looking for? She surmised that she must be half asleep, so she went back to bed. The feeling persisted, so once again she went around the room and this time she noticed the postcard which was ready to be mailed. She sensed that her search had something to do with it. Gloria sat back on her bed and asked God that if He was in this, He'd have to tell her what to look for. She thought that maybe she should put a sticker on the card to brighten it up a bit, but she knew that her box of stickers had been lost for many weeks. She had almost taken her apartment apart looking for them when she needed them for the cradle roll for her church, but had been unable to find them.

By now, while sitting on her bed, her feet were getting cold so she bent down to get her slippers. There was only one there, so assuming that the other one had been pushed under the bed, she took her crutch and swung it under the bed. Out came the slipper and the lost box of stickers. On top was a sheet of very plain stickers with Bible verses on them. She immediately put that sheet to the bottom of the pile as they were too drab to brighten up the card. She had many beautiful stickers in that box, but she didn't feel right about any of them. Finally she went back to the first sheet, and even though she did not like those, she felt she should use one of them. She asked God to help her pick the right verse. She ripped off the first one, but at the last moment she put it on another letter that was also ready to be mailed. She thought the next one must be the one, but it tore in half instead of along the perforations. The third one was the sticker she put on my postcard. She had no idea why, but she sensed that it was the one the Lord wanted her to use.

I was absolutely amazed. When we were going through Merv's burnout and my breast cancer, we knew God was with us by faith because He promises to never leave us or forsake us (Josh. 1:5). He had not done anything awesome to strengthen our faith, but now He had done this! God's ways surely are higher than our ways (Isaiah 55:8-9), and I do not try to understand when, how or why He chooses to reveal Himself.

On Monday morning, three weeks before Christmas, I was called to teach for a day, and that day stretched into three weeks. The teacher was in the hospital, and I was told that the job might continue for a while after the holidays. What a blessing! Instead of having to wait for the phone to ring each morning to find out if and where I would be teaching that day, I knew where I would be. Since I was very busy with eight classes every day, I had no time to get depressed about my upcoming surgery, so it was easy to stay in my "box for today." We put up our tree; Anita and I still insisted it would be a good Christmas.

᠊ᠬᠵᠬᠵᠬ᠊

A few days before my surgery, we invited two elders and their wives for supper. They anointed me with oil and prayed for a successful operation and healing. I told them about the postcard from Gloria and we all rejoiced. God's peace was with us in full measure.

On the morning of my surgery, we all felt very positive. We dropped Anita off at the home of her friend Annette, so they could do some last minute Christmas shopping, and Merv and I went to the hospital. I had total peace as I waited in a little room in the day surgery department. I was eventually called, and while I was on the stretcher wearing a silly hospital gown, a nurse asked if I had been in Florida. When I replied that I had not, she said I looked tanned. I knew it was my dark complexion that had fooled her.

I was given the anesthesia, and the next thing I knew I was waking up in the recovery room. I was so glad it was over and the warmed blankets that were wrapped around me were very comforting. Soon the surgeon came to talk to me. He had a big smile on his face as he told me that the lump in my breast was a fibrous mass, definitely not malignant. The shoulder lump appeared to be some kind of a cyst, and again, no sign of any malignancy. He told me to go home and enjoy a great Christmas. I thanked him and said, "So that's the verdict. No cancer." He replied that because the lab reports were not available, he couldn't say with complete certainly, but he would say that he was ninety-nine per cent sure there was no cancer. I knew that the doctor had a very good reputation for being accurate in his diagnoses, so ninety-nine per cent was excellent. I got dressed and met Merv in the waiting room with a huge smile on my face. It was fantastic to meet him with good news for a change. I went to bed for the rest of the day and it was a blessing to be home. After supper I phoned several friends from church to share the good news. I also phoned my parents and other family members. They decided to delay the Christmas dinner until after I would be able to make the trip, as I was to see the surgeon in a week.

We had a wonderful, quiet Christmas Day, thankful that all four of us were healthy.

≈ 20 ≈

*T*he appointment for the post-operative checkup was made for December 29. I asked for a very early time as we would be leaving for the family Christmas celebrations in the Kitchener area immediately afterwards. I was told the surgeon would be in the hospital in a small town close to Ottawa in the morning. Since that was on our way, I arranged to see him there. On the morning of the 29th, we packed all our things in the car and the four of us set off. Anita and I had been right after all—it *was* a good Christmas!

When we arrived at the hospital Dave decided to go in with me because he dislikes waiting in the car for any length of time. He joked that there would be more leg room in the waiting room than in the car. Merv had to find a bank machine, and Anita went with him. I knew that this appointment would be over quickly as both my incisions had healed very well.

Soon I was called and was once again told to "strip from the waist up." When the surgeon came in and asked about my Christmas, I assured him that it had been super. I told him that we were going to visit with the extended family. He asked when, and I replied, "Right now. Merv and the kids are waiting for me." A strange look crossed his face as he started telling me that he had the lab reports. The breast lump was indeed benign, but he was sorry to say that the shoulder lump was malignant. In fact, it was a metastasis of the kidney cancer. I just put my face in my hands and whispered, "Oh God." I thought of the seven months that were lost due to the lipoma misdiagnosis! He went on to say that everyone was absolutely shocked. No one had suspected that it was malignant. The pathologist was so astounded that he personally phoned the surgeon, who in turn phoned the urologist to tell him. He too was very shocked. Obviously I wasn't the only one who had difficulty believing this news. He said he had been informed before Christmas, but he just didn't have the heart to tell me. I thanked him. I wondered how the cancer could have moved from my left kidney to my right shoulder, and he confirmed my suspicions—it must have traveled in my blood.

So that was it. I had renal cell cancer in my blood! Where else had it gone? I looked him straight in the eye and said, "You've just given me my death sentence, haven't you?" He thought for a moment, then replied, "Not necessarily." He went on to say that I would be having many tests and then we would know more. I shared with him that I was not afraid to die and that many people were praying for me. The remainder of that conversation did not mean very much to me, because all I could think about was how I would tell Merv and the kids that I had kidney cancer again.

We all knew how life threatening it would be if that disease spread.

Somehow I got dressed and when Dave saw me coming down the hall, he jumped up and we walked through the first set of doors that led to the main entrance. We looked out and saw that Merv and Anita had not yet returned, so there between the two sets of doors I told Dave. I'm five feet tall and he is six feet, so he looked down at me, put his arm around me and said, "What are we going to do with this little Mommy of ours?" I knew he was hurting too. Soon the car drove up and we got in. I told Merv and Anita. Her reaction was predictable. She was quiet. Merv, for the first time, started crying, sobbing as if his heart would break. My tears came too. We made a quick decision to continue on the trip, but we seemed to be a family totally different from the happy, carefree one that had been in the car half an hour earlier.

As we drove off, Merv suggested that we all pray out loud. He and I took our turns, but the kids were silent. I knew they were praying, but the moment was far too tense for them to share their innermost thoughts. By the time we got to Perth we decided to phone an elder so the prayer chain could be started once again. We knew we would need massive amounts of prayer, especially over the next few days. After all, we were on the way to celebrate a family Christmas. Merv made the call from a pay phone, and when he returned to the car, he said that Pat said to tell me that she loved me. My tears came again, as she was one of the friends I had phoned just a week earlier to tell her the good news after the surgery. I also made a call from the phone booth to my friend Christa. She would hear about it on the prayer chain, but I wanted to share it with her personally. She was not home so I left a message on the answering machine. Have you ever left that kind of message? It was very difficult, but I assured her that I would be all right because God was with us.

The rest of the five and a half hours of our trip was very long and very quiet. As we traveled I happened to notice that the palms of my hands had a yellow tinge. In fact the back of my hands did too. I remembered the nurse who had asked if I had been in Florida. My whole body must be yellow. Terror struck! It had spread to my liver! I prayed constantly but said nothing to anyone about my discovery.

We finally arrived at my parents' home, put on our fake smiles and said nothing about my health. Later, we went to my brother's home. After the kids went to bed, we shared our news as we sat around the table in their big farm kitchen. We were honest and let them know just how serious this was. They too entered into the shock and pain with us.

When we finally got into bed I was exhausted, but I knew that sleep would not come easily. During all the other crises, God had blessed me with the ability to sleep. The few times I couldn't, I would get my tape player and listen to a tape called "Springs of Comfort." By the time the tape had ended, God's peace was back and I would fall asleep. There I was—in my worst crisis, in a strange bed, without my tapes and tracts that had given me so much comfort in the past. I read my Bible, and Merv and I prayed together—and individually—but we spent a very restless night.

The next morning I phoned my sister and again, even though the words were coming out of my mouth, it seemed impossible that this was really happening. We decided that I needed to tell my dad, but until we knew more, we would not say anything to my mother. She seemed to be fighting nerve problems and this information would not help her recovery. That morning I waited for a chance to talk privately with Dad. When he and I were alone in the kitchen, I motioned for him to come into the basement. He sat down, and as gently but truthfully as possible, I explained the situation to him. He just looked down at the floor, wringing his hands. I told him we all thought that Mom couldn't handle this news and I wondered if he agreed.

Without looking up, he replied, "That's right. Don't tell her. But how am I going to handle it?" There, in that basement room, my 82-year-old father was grieving for me. I felt awful that I had told him, and yet I knew I had to.

We went into town later that morning. I decided to buy some non-prescription sleeping pills, in case I would have another night when sleeping was difficult. I felt maybe that was a lack of faith so I did much soul searching before I bought them. I'm not sure why I felt like that, since I would take an aspirin any time for a headache without even thinking about it. That night, just knowing they were there helped greatly. When I got home they were not needed at all.

The time for dinner and opening gifts arrived, and in spite of everything, we had a very jolly time. The only difficult moment for me was at the table when I began to wonder if I would be there next year. Probably everyone except my mom had those same thoughts at some time during the meal.

Dave took the bus home to Ottawa on New Year's Eve day and Anita was invited to see the new year in with a friend in Stratford. My brother and his wife had also been invited out. Merv and I had decided to stay by ourselves even though some friends in Waterloo had asked us to spend the evening with them. We didn't think we'd want to celebrate. As night approached and darkness descended we began to think that being alone was not very wise, so we phoned our friends and asked if we could still come. They said they would be delighted to have us. We had a wonderful time greeting the new year. Again I realized how important an invitation to hurting people can be. We all knew we had a rough road ahead of us in 1993, but with the Lord's help, we could face whatever was in store. That year was to be another one spent in the Valley of the Shadow of Cancer.

❧ 21 ❧

*T*he trip home was a very welcome one. It would be good to be home with my tapes and tracts and close to our church family whom we knew were praying for us. When I was asked to continue in that teaching job, I told the principal that my health problems would require some time off for tests. I had the job for six more weeks and in that time missed only one and a half days.

My first appointment was with the radiation oncologist whom I had been seeing since my bout with breast cancer. He immediately asked me when I found out "this bad news." I told him about the seven months that were lost due to the misdiagnosis of the lump. He felt that in cases like this the later one found out the better. It was obvious that even though he was not a renal cell cancer specialist, he certainly was aware of how deadly this was.

He had me disrobe. First he asked if I wanted Merv to stay in the room and I said I did. He had never been in an examining room with me before, but I really needed him there just for support. The doctor ran his hands over my whole body and found no other lumps. (It was embarrassing to have Merv there, so in subsequent appointments I have not asked him to remain for my examinations.) I showed the doctor a tiny lump I had recently discovered on my knee, but he was not interested in it. He said only that I should keep an eye on it. He probably thought I would be dead long before that lump could cause any problems.

❧❧

He told us that between one and two per cent of people who have a metastasis of kidney cancer survive. Instead of being destroyed, I was encouraged by those words. That's called God's grace! He continued by saying that since it had taken several years for the lump to show, my cancer seemed to be slow in progressing. Things might not be *quite* as bad as they looked.

Merv asked the oncologist about my "yellow" skin. I was so glad that he asked because I did not have the courage to mention it. The doctor laughed and pointed to the bright yellow walls in the tiny examining room. He thought we all looked yellow, but Merv then explained that I always have a yellow tinge. Finally I told him that I thought it had spread to my liver. He said I could check by taking a mirror outside, or having Merv look into my eyes in daylight. If the whites of my eyes were white, it was not a liver problem. I don't need to say that Merv checked my eyes as soon as we went through the exit doors of the hospital. They were white! Thank you Lord!

When I told Dave about the survival rate, he said, "You're shooting for that two per cent, aren't you Mom?" I assured him I was. My teaching continued and I enjoyed every minute at school.

My next appointment was with the holistic doctor. He was well aware of how grave my situation was, but he was very willing to help me fight it. As he is also a Christian, we both knew that God would have the final say in my healing, but I would do whatever *I* could. The doctor increased some of the dosages, removed some items and added others. When I asked what the difference was between what I had been taking and what I would be taking now, his reply was, "You were driving a Chev, now you're driving a Rolls." I am still driving that Rolls and will probably do so as long as I live. These are immune system boosters and it appears that my immune system needs lots of help. Additionally, I was told to have meat only three times a week and to eat massive amounts of fresh vegetables. I mentioned my yellow color and he had the answer. It was caused by all the beta carotene I was taking. So now I joke about my beta carotene tan when someone comments about my skin colour.

Those appointments were relatively easy, but then came the time for the tests. I was going to have blood work done, chest x-rays, an extensive ultrasound and a bone scan. Knowing that there was almost nothing that medical science could do for me, I made the decision that I would not have the bone scan. That test involved an injection of radioactive fluid—not something that would benefit my depressed immune system, which already had had five weeks of radiation to deal with the year before. I didn't see the value of that procedure at all. I phoned the kidney cancer specialist whom I had not yet met. She admitted that even if they would find cancer in my bones, there was nothing they could do. She asked about my health in general and if I was experiencing any bone aches. When I replied that I was feeling fine, teaching everyday and had no pain in my bones, she said that the bone scan probably was not necessary.

I have learned not to blindly do everything doctors recommend. If I feel uncomfortable about something, I pray about it and then do whatever I think the Holy Spirit is leading me to do.

∽◈∾

The day of the tests was tense. The ultrasound was first, and since it was early morning I could not have breakfast prior to it. Merv and I promised ourselves a big, unhealthy breakfast of bacon, eggs, homefries and coffee after the test. Those foods were on my forbidden list, so it would be a very special meal.

We arrived at the hospital after a quiet drive. Even though God's peace was there, it was a trying day. Soon I was on the examining table. I had had ultrasounds before, but I realized that this one was different. It was taking so long! I thought of Merv. He had never had to wait that long before.

I never look at the screen during this procedure because everything looks like a tumor to the untrained eye. I also do not watch the technician's face, as I would probably read a lot into her expression. Usually I just lie there, eyes shut, praying. That is what I was doing, but as the time dragged on I got scared. What was she seeing on the monitor? I was tempted to look, but did not. I knew that my consultation concerning the results of all the tests was scheduled for late afternoon and I couldn't imagine waiting that long. I prayed that if everything was O.K. (which I doubted at that point), God would prompt her to give me a hint about it. Then I realized that if she said nothing (which is what they are supposed to do), having prayed that prayer, I would be convinced that something *was* wrong. I had prayed myself into a corner! I prayed again, this time asking God to forget my previous request as it would be better if she said nothing. Little did that technician realize the dialogue that was going on between that room and heaven! Well, God gave grace and finally she said, "You may go now, Mrs. Bouwman. I have checked everything and it all looks good." I cautiously asked if that meant she did not see anything abnormal, and she replied, "That's right." (Thank you Lord for answering my first prayer even though I had canceled it!)

Merv and I had a long, delicious breakfast as we rejoiced with the wonderful news that all my organs were free of tumors.

The next tests were the blood work and chest x-rays. Even though we were still facing the consultation and the results of those tests, I felt as if an unbelievable weight had been lifted from my shoulders since the news of the ultrasound. That made the wait for the consultation more bearable.

At last my name was called. Merv's eyes met mine and I knew that he was tense too. Sometimes it is harder for the loved ones than for the patient.

I was greeted in the small room by a very young medical student. When he started checking my eyes and ears I just couldn't keep quiet any longer. "You're not looking for kidney cancer in my eyes and ears, are you?" I asked. He blushed and admitted that he was doing a routine physical. It took him a long time, but eventually the specialist came in. She wanted to see how he had examined my organs so he had to repeat most of what he had just done, this time explaining to her what he was doing. Didn't these two realize that I was very anxious to get the test results, which would either be a death sentence or a new lease on life?

After what seemed like an eternity, I was allowed to get dressed and then Merv was sent in. We waited for the doctor to return. Eventually she and the student came in with a huge file. She told us what we already knew about the ultrasound and then added that the blood tests and chest x-ray were fine. There was no evidence of cancer anywhere!

This news was almost too good to totally comprehend. I think in situations like that, most people brace themselves for the worst, so it takes a while to realize that the imminent crisis had passed. She stressed that a few people do survive for as long as ten years. She predicted that I would continue to develop tumors, but as long as they avoided my major organs, surgery would control the disease. She said nothing about being rid of it permanently. I showed her the tiny lump on my knee, but she just said it should be watched. When I asked about my teaching, she replied, "Never put your life on hold for something like this." At that point the student piped up, saying that there was a cyst on one of my ovaries. That was scary, and never having had one before, I asked what would be done about it. The doctor suggested that my family physician should follow it. Sometimes they disappeared, and other times they grew large and had to be surgically removed. I couldn't believe what I was hearing. I wondered if it was really a cyst or was this another instance of misdiagnosis? The mention of surgery sent shock waves through my entire system. With God's help, Merv and I decided to rejoice with the good news and forget about the cyst for the time being. After all, if surgery would be necessary, it was not in our "box for today"! We went home and phoned family and friends, telling them our wonderful news. We said nothing about my ovarian cyst.

⁊◦⊱

My teaching continued and I had a heart full of thanksgiving all the time. Even though I had a very slim chance of surviving, at present I was well.

In a few weeks I had my initial visit with my new family doctor. She did a physical and reviewed my medical history. She had received the reports from the Cancer Clinic, so I asked about the cyst. She read the report to me and said that in about two months she would book another ultrasound to check it. I wondered if it was indeed a cyst. She assured me that ultrasounds are very accurate in distinguishing between solid masses and cysts. I decided to believe that, even though so many other mistakes had been made before. After the Pap test I was on my way. I liked my new doctor and felt happy that she seemed to be credible.

After some time I received a phone call from her office. The nurse was very gentle and started by telling me that the doctor wanted to make sure that I would not think that this phone call meant that I had cancer. My heart sank. She went on to say that my Pap test results were questionable, so I was to come in for another one. Apparently, this happens quite frequently, and usually the follow-up test is negative. I was told very strongly not to worry as it probably was nothing. After all I had gone through, it took some determination, as well as a fresh supply of God's grace, to be able to be free from worry. The repeat test was scheduled, and before I had the results, I had the ultrasound to check my ovarian cyst. Merv always goes with me when I have tests, but I went by myself because I knew I wouldn't find out anything anyway. I arrived at the clinic with a very full bladder as I had to drink a lot of fluid prior to the test.

I was told to strip, and then the technician came in. It soon became obvious that she was not only checking my ovary, in fact she was checking *all* my organs, especially the uterus. She kept on going back to that area and then started asking questions like, "When was your last period? How many pregnancies did you have? When was your last Pap test?" That last question freaked me out, as I did not have the results of the last test, and the previous one was questionable. What was on that monitor to make her ask those questions? I felt devastated. This ultrasound was even worse than the big one several weeks earlier. At least I had braced myself for bad news. This time I was completely unprepared.

I prayed while she called in another technician. I did not want to hear what they said. I knew I would read doom and gloom into any comments they made, so as I lay on my side, my one ear was against the pillow and I blocked the other with my finger. I hoped they wouldn't notice but I just couldn't listen to their conversation. Well, it worked—so well that when they asked me to take a deep breath I did not hear them. After saying it three times, they shook me to get my attention. I had to admit why I hadn't heard, and for a moment my embarrassment was greater than my fear. When the second technician left the room I was told I could go.

In a daze I found a small washroom and emptied my ready-to-burst bladder. Then I went back to the little cubicle where my clothing was. When I got into my car, the tears came. I was convinced that she had found a tumor in my uterus. I cried for awhile, dried my tears and drove home. I decided not to tell anyone about this experience. I just did not have the strength to share any more bad news and besides, there was always a chance that all was well. But, in truth, I doubted that.

≈≈≈

That week I spent a lot of time in prayer, and although I had peace, there was a heaviness present. Again, I remembered Bea's words: "It never ends." Finally the phone rang. It was my doctor's nurse. My heart raced and my throat got dry when I heard her voice. She said that she had the results of the ultrasound, indicating that the cyst had disappeared and all the other organs were normal. She also had the results of the second Pap test, and it was fine. This was too good to be true. I was very thankful, but also very confused. Why did I have to have the second Pap test? Why had that technician asked all those questions when everything was fine? At times like this I am very aware that God's ways are not our ways (Isaiah 55:8-9). He could have had a negative test result on the first Pap test, and He could have had the cyst disappear before the first ultrasound. Then I would have been spared all that extra stress. I was thankful that I had been able to conquer most of my worries, but those concerns were in the back of my mind during that time of waiting. I believed God had a purpose, so I accepted it and continued to pray that whatever I was to learn from this, I would learn quickly. Once again I resolved to live in my "box for today"!

On my next visit to the surgeon I showed him the tiny lump on my knee and one I had just discovered on my arm. He decided to do a biopsy, even though he was very certain that they both were lipomas. This time I did not worry at all. I asked God to be in control, and by His grace I refused to think about it. The biopsies were done at the hospital with local anesthesia. As the surgeon removed them he was happy to report that they were lipomas. They would be sent to the lab and I would have the official report within a week. There seemed to be a touch of déjà vu in all of that, but I was not fearful. I was in and out of the hospital in twenty-five minutes.

Merv and I joked that my hospital stays seemed to be developing an encouraging trend. For the initial kidney surgery, I was in the hospital eighteen days. For my breast cancer surgery, my stay was three days. I was in the hospital about three hours for the removal of the breast and shoulder lumps. Now I was out in twenty-five minutes! We hoped this meant there would be no more hospital stays of any duration in the near future.

In a week I received the report that both lumps were indeed lipomas and therefore not malignant. Even though I had absolutely not worried, I heaved a big sigh of relief and gratefulness that God had once again protected me. I soon had the stitches removed, and compared with my other incisions, they were very insignificant. Life in the Valley of the Shadow of Cancer certainly has its ups and downs, but the good news is that our Heavenly Father is there at all times.

∽ 22 ∾

Since I had no lumps or bumps left and all my regular tests had come back negative, we had planned to have a relaxing summer '93, enjoying our home and my good health.

My father had begun to exhibit strange symptoms in March and April, including a drooping lip, which was still evident in late July when he developed double vision. When he was hospitalized I went to their home to care for my mother, who was rapidly developing numerous signs of dementia. After many tests my father was told he had a brain tumor. Merv and I took him to see a neurosurgeon in London. As we sat with Dad in the waiting area, it all seemed very strange. I had battled two cancers that are notorious for spreading to the brain and now there we were, waiting with my father who had a brain tumor. As this was the first day the surgeon was back after his holidays, our wait stretched into several hours. The surgeon was overbooked and overworked. Finally, he came in with the MRI and CAT scan reports. As I looked at the image of the tumor, I couldn't help but wonder if this was God's way of introducing me to this very skilled brain surgeon. Would I be needing his services some day? After examining my dad, he decided that the tumor was not the source of his problems. He felt that it was a benign tumor that had probably been there for years. Dad was admitted to the hospital that night. His one eye could no longer close, so the concern was that he would lose his sight.

As we left the hospital we were handed a booklet for brain tumor patients and their families. I paged through it and discovered that it was dedicated to a patient who had died of a brain tumor—a metastasis of kidney cancer! (Lord, do I really need to be going through this?)

~≈~

That summer turned out to be a very difficult one. My mother was put into respite care in a nursing home. We went back and forth several times, and in September my father passed away. God allowed me to be with him just minutes before he died. I had arrived by bus from Ottawa at 5:00 p.m. I fed him supper and then sat by his bedside and prayed. At 6:00 p.m., I told him that since I had been on the bus all day I was hungry. I asked if I should go for supper then, or wait until he fell asleep. He said I should go then, so before I left for the cafeteria I squeezed his hand and said, "I'll be back soon. I love you." Those were the last words ever spoken to him. When I arrived back in his room half an hour later, he had passed away in his sleep. He had not moved a finger since I had left him. He had just peacefully gone home to be with his Lord. I called a nurse. His death was confirmed with a stethoscope.

We knew he was very ill, but no one, not even the nurses, suspected he was that close to death. This was a shock, but beautiful peace surrounded everything. I called Merv and the rest of the family. I had put together all my clothes that I would need for the funeral in case Dad would die, so

I reminded Merv to bring that clothing bag along the next day. Again I wondered why I had been the one to be with Dad during his last minutes on earth, and why I was the first to find him after he had passed away. Was God preparing me to face my own death?

For my brother and his wife this was an especially hard time, because within twelve weeks of my dad's death, my sister-in-law's parents passed away.

Through all the stress and late nights I felt fine, and we continued to thank God for His gift of good health.

∞ 23 ∞

On returning home, I was informed that my oncologist had moved to a different hospital so my next appointment had been transferred to that hospital. It turned out to be the most frustrating hospital appointment to date. I mention it to encourage others in the Valley when they have similar experiences. They need to know they are not alone in dealing with frustrating and uncontrollable events.

Because it was my first visit to that hospital, I did not have a blue card. I was directed to where I could get one. We have a long address—street number, post office box number, and rural route number. The lady had a hard time fitting all that information on the little card. Several times she tried, but the machine that prints the cards would not accept her format. Finally, we both worked on it, shortening every word possible. She came back looking very frustrated. The machine had accepted it, but had run out of cards, and the format was lost. We tried to remember how we had set it up, and at last I had the card in my hand.

I left that area and returned to the waiting room where Merv was reading a magazine to pass the time. I had to go to the end of a long line and when I finally got to the receptionist, she took the blue card and told me to sit down until the doctor was ready to see me. By now almost an hour had passed and as I sat there, I realized that she had not said anything about the tests I always had. I stood in line again and awaited my turn. I asked the receptionist when I was to have my tests and after looking over the requisition, she said there were none scheduled. I told her that I always had chest x-rays and blood work done half an hour before the consultation. She insisted that I was not to have any tests. I went back to Merv. He went to a pay phone to ask the other Cancer Clinic personnel. My file was checked, and he was told that I certainly was to have the tests.

I stood in line once again and told the woman what Merv had found out, but she would not budge. I returned to Merv and we were both thoroughly frustrated and disgusted with the system. Then I remembered that I had my appointment card from the other clinic in my purse. Since the last appointment had been rescheduled, the card should solve the problem. It read, "Tests—1:00 p.m., Consultation—1:30 p.m." I took it to the receptionist, and this time I refused to go to the back of the line. All she said was that she couldn't do anything about it. I would have to discuss it with my doctor. Again I went back to Merv and we began to wonder if we would ever get out of that place.

Finally my name was called and I was told to "strip from the waist up." I sat on the examining table and waited again. After a long time a young doctor who I had never seen came in. I couldn't believe my ears when she started back at square one with questions like, "Has anyone in your family ever had cancer?" I was polite, but inside I was screaming, "I've had it three times! Does it really matter if any of my relatives had it?!" She finally examined my breasts, and it would not have surprised me if that was her first time. I thought I would probably have to have a lump the size of an orange for her to find it. When she finished, she said that I was fine and could go. I told her that I had not had my tests. When she said there were none scheduled, I jumped off the table, grabbed my purse, and as graciously as I could, showed her the card that stated the time for the tests. She too said that there was nothing she could do, so I suggested that she should ask the oncologist since he was the one who had scheduled them at the other hospital. I knew that he was there as I had seen him through the door when she came in. She reluctantly left the room and again I had to wait. She returned saying that the oncologist said it would be all right. I could have the tests when I would come back in four months! We had spent over three hours in that hospital and had learned absolutely nothing about the state of my health. To add insult to injury, the parking fee was $10.00! We quickly made the decision to go back to the other Cancer Clinic, even though it meant a new oncologist.

❧ 24 ❧

In October '93, I celebrated my 50th birthday. I considered that a milestone, since I was only 45-years-old when I first entered the Valley. Merv and the kids planned a surprise party, and I was amazed at how naive I had been. Never once did I suspect anything. It was wonderful to celebrate with the people whose prayers had been instrumental in my recovery.

In a short while it was time to make Christmas plans. Since there were no tests scheduled before the holidays, and I was feeling fine, Anita and I once again talked about having a good Christmas. She had started college in September, so with the exception of some weekends, Merv and I were empty nesters. We were looking forward to having both kids home over the holidays. We had a wonderful time together and were very thankful for my good health. We traveled to the extended family celebrations, and as we sat around the table for the Christmas dinner my thoughts wandered to the previous year's meal. I had thought that I would perhaps be the missing one, but instead it was Dad. In fact, we had an extra person that year. My niece and her husband had had a baby boy on December 8, so little Trevor was the highlight of the gathering. That helped ease the pain of Dad's absence. We celebrated the new year, and hoped that 1994 would be a year of good health.

≫◦≪

Supply teaching kept me very busy, and we continued to redecorate our home. I faithfully took all the vitamins that the holistic doctor had been prescribing, and I was very careful with what I ate. I also continued to have my time with the Lord first thing most mornings. My friends and family were still praying for me.

On my next Cancer Clinic appointment I met my new oncologist. He reviewed my case and told me that I should know that some people do survive a metastasis of kidney cancer. I said that I knew it was between one and two per cent, and he agreed. Then he came very close to saying that I might be one of them. Apparently it is very unusual to go a whole year without any more tumors. He seemed pleased. I was very happy to share his words with Merv and the kids.

We had a lovely summer. Merv and I took several short trips to visit relatives and friends. We also had the sale of my parents' property, so that chapter in our lives has been closed. In late August I had my regular Cancer Clinic appointment. My oncologist was very pleased with my health. I was relieved to hear that a new fluctuating lump that I had found in my breast was no problem. Changing lumps are almost always benign. Before he left the room he shook my hand and said, "Congratulations! Whatever you're doing, you're doing it right." I told him that what I was doing was "lots of prayer and lots of vitamins." I make it a point to tell my doctors how vital my faith is in coping with this disease.

✎ 25 ✎

*A*s usual fall was a wonderful season, and my health was excellent. Eventually we began making plans for Christmas '94. Anita and I once again said it would be a good holiday season. In early December, I finished this book, and was waiting for Anita to complete the typing. It was an ideal place to end—two years cancer free!

My next appointment was scheduled for December 22— three days before Christmas. I was tempted to cancel it and reschedule it for January because of the bad news I had received before other Christmases, but I decided to keep it since I was in excellent health.

✎✎

On December 22, Anita and I went into the city to do some last minute shopping. We met Merv and together we went to the Cancer Clinic. Anita went with us. She would be graduating in a few months from her Medical Office Administration course, and her job might be at that hospital.

The tests were over quickly, and I had no apprehension whatsoever. Soon I was called into the examining room and when I once again had "stripped from the waist up," a young doctor whom I had never met before, entered. She introduced herself, said that she had just read my file, and then immediately started talking about that lump. I told her that it was still fluctuating. I also mentioned that I had had many breast lumps in the past. She then asked if I had ever seriously considered having both breasts removed!

I said I had not. I couldn't believe the insensitivity of this person. She had known me for all of two minutes, and had the nerve to ask me that question with as much emotion as one would ask about the weather. I thought it was grossly inappropriate and dismissed it immediately.

Then she said that I should not show her where the lump was—she wanted to see if she could find it herself. She checked and asked if it was the little one that felt like a pea. I didn't even know I had a lump in my breast that felt like a pea. Somehow there was something very wrong about this appointment. When I finally showed her the other lump, she said she would get the oncologist to check it. He came in, examined me and asked if there had been a needle biopsy done. When I told him there hadn't, he said he would like to do one immediately. Was I hearing correctly? I reminded him that four months before, he had thought that lump was okay. I told him I knew that my surgeon did not have much faith in needle biopsies. The oncologist said the procedure would be good because, if it came back positive, we would know for sure. I couldn't believe this! He sounded quite certain that it was malignant, although he didn't exactly say that.

I told him (with a throat that by now was very dry) that since it was three days before Christmas, I did not want the needle biopsy. Instead I would go to the surgeon right after the holidays. He said that would be okay—after all, if the results were positive I would need to see the surgeon anyway, and if they were negative he would send me there for a second opinion. When he said he was concerned because the lump was above the incision, I knew he must have found a new one because the other one was below. I again assured him that I would see the surgeon right after Christmas, and the young doctor informed me that they would send him a letter "today." I had the feeling that those two doctors knew something I didn't. They left the room and I got dressed in a daze. Merv and Anita were waiting and I quickly told them that I needed to see the surgeon immediately after Christmas. I tried to be upbeat, but I couldn't hide my shock. My next appointment was booked for March, and I noticed that on my appointment card there were no tests scheduled. I told the secretary I always had tests, so she checked with the oncologist. He said there were to be none. Why? I was afraid to ask. I was convinced that he thought I would be hospitalized for breast cancer surgery, so those tests would be redundant. I felt as though I was trying to think through a fog, and as the three of us walked out of the revolving door of the Cancer Clinic, I realized that neither doctor had told me the results of the chest x-ray that had just been taken. Since they always had in the past, I was terrified, but I decided not to say anything, nor to go back and ask. I did not need more bad news three days before Christmas.

Merv suggested we stop at the surgeon's office, but I refused. In a few minutes he asked again, reminding me that not knowing is often worse than knowing. This time I agreed, but when we arrived at his office the door was locked. Was God protecting me from even worse news?

Merv dropped Anita and me off at the mall, and with heavy hearts we quickly finished our shopping. On the way home we talked about the appointment and she said, "I guess God wants a few more chapters in your book." She was right. The ending I had just written needed to be scrapped; there was more to write. (Oh God, how much more?) Then in silence my mind raced. I reasoned that if something had showed up on the chest x-ray, the oncologist would have sent me to the surgeon. Instead, I had been the one who had suggested that I go. Also, since December marked the third year since my breast cancer, and two years since my metastasis, maybe my tests would be every six months from now on. Maybe everything would be okay....

When we arrived home we quickly stoked up the fire in the woodstove, put on Christmas music and turned on the tree lights. I prayed a short prayer, and peace filled my soul as the warmth from the fire warmed the house as well as our shattered emotions. I told Anita that we would not be talking or thinking about the appointment until after Christmas. It was not in our box for those days! Merv telephoned the surgeon's office later that day and made an appointment. I was very glad he had done that, for then I knew that nothing would happen until January 5. That night I checked my breast. I could hardly find the fluctuating lump, but there was one above the incision. It felt like a cyst.

Dave arrived with Anita's boyfriend the next afternoon, and we had some wonderful days together. Christmas was perfect. Our concerns about cancer would just have to wait!

Merv and I traveled to spend several days with our extended family right after Christmas. We shared with them my upcoming visit with the surgeon. We did not let that spoil our time together, but on New Year's Eve, we couldn't help wondering what lay ahead in 1995 as we continued our journey in the Valley.

✎ 26 ✎

Since I would not be teaching until the schools reopened on January 9, 1995, Merv took time off work until then too. The kids were back at their schools and Merv and I had a very special time—sleeping in, sitting by the fire, spending time with the Lord, and reading. Much of our reading was about the connection between diet and degenerative diseases, including cancer. We were encouraged and excited by what we read. My diet was very good, but it still needed some improvement. Instead of limiting my intake of foods such as white flour, sugar, refined oils, fried foods, coffee, meat and all other animal products, I realized that these needed to be removed completely from my diet.

One night as I was preparing for bed I discovered a new lump. It was small (the size of a pea), just under the skin on my rib cage, about an inch below the breast that had previously had cancer. (The other lumps were in the other breast.) I showed Merv and he thought it was just part of the bone, but when I felt it as I lay in different positions, I knew it was not just the bone.

On January 5, we reluctantly went to the surgeon. I showed him the new lump on my rib cage first. He checked it but said nothing. He then examined the other breast. He said he still had no problem with the fluctuating lump, as it probably was a ridge resulting from the last biopsy two years earlier. He then found three cysts and aspirated them. That included the ones the oncologists had been concerned about. It is always such a relief to see the liquid being drawn into the needle. He was quite satisfied that all was well in that breast. The oncologists had been wrong!

Then he checked the new lump on my rib cage once again, but this time he said it had to come out. He did not seem overly concerned, but considering that the lump on my shoulder had proved cancerous against his expectations, he wanted to investigate this one. He would use local anesthetic, so I would be in and out of the hospital in about half an hour. I had absolutely no fear. I think I would have been very upset if I had needed general anesthesia, but somehow this did not seem as much like another operation. I was booked in for January 20, and was told that it might be sooner if they had a cancellation. We went home and continued praying and reading our books. On Monday, the biopsy was moved up to January 13, only four days away. I was relieved that the wait had been shortened.

The next evening as I was undressing to take a shower, I

noticed in the mirror that the lump was very visible when I lifted my arm. It seemed to stick out, and it looked larger than I had thought. When I bent in different directions I could see and feel that it did not move with the skin. In fact, it seemed to be attached to the ribs. That was very frightening. My soapy fingers explored it dozens of times as I showered.

When I returned to the family room, I felt abandoned. Merv was there, the flames in the woodstove were dancing and my favorite tape was playing, but sorrow overwhelmed me. The last straw was when my eyes happened to glance over at the pictures of my niece's two darling little children. These were my brother's grandchildren and at that moment any hopes of my being alive to see my own grandchildren someday were shattered. The tears came. I tried to hide them from Merv, but couldn't. For several minutes I sobbed the heart-wrenching sobs of a person who had lost all hope. Apparently those tears were very therapeutic, because when I finally dried my red eyes, I felt refreshed and hope slowly seeped back into my barren soul. Grandchildren were not in my box for that night!

❧❧

The morning of my biopsy arrived—Friday the 13th. I was very thankful that I am not superstitious. Before we left, I asked God to give me a verse from my "Promise Box"—a word from Him for that day. I don't usually do that, but even though I had no fear, I felt very vulnerable. I chose a little card from the middle of the box. I was delighted with the verse—Psalm 34:19: "Many are the afflictions of the righteous, but the Lord delivers him out of them all"(NKJV). I realized that death might be His way of delivering me, but the verse gave me peace anyway. I stuck it into my pocket and off we went. As we were entering the hospital Merv asked how I felt. I said that I thought I should be "baaing." I did not need to explain that I felt like a lamb being led to the slaughter.

The wait was short and soon I was in a small room being asked once again to "strip from the waist up." The surgeon injected the local anesthetic and began his task. It took longer than he had expected and he needed to give me a second shot when I began to feel him "digging." He apologized and said that it was deeper than he had anticipated. That didn't surprise me since I had discovered that it seemed to be attached to the rib.

When he was done, he said that it was yellowish and that he did not know what it was. The fact that it was yellow sort of made me chuckle. I thought that with all the beta carotene I was taking, my blood would soon take on a yellow tinge too! As I left I realized that he had said nothing either encouraging or discouraging. Another wait for test results was just beginning. That evening we were invited to Pat and Frank's for dinner. They realized that we would need some encouragement. Again an invitation at just the right time was a blessing.

During that next week I continued to read the books on cancer, nutrition and alternate therapies, and improved my diet. I also spent a lot of time with the Lord, both in my quiet time and on my walks which had become a daily activity. I prayed for my own healing and that of several others who had recently had cancer diagnoses. The tapes that had ministered to me in my other cancer crises once again helped keep my mind in "perfect peace"(Is. 26:3). Due to the tenderness of my incision, I had to sleep on my right side or on my back. Since I always sleep on my left side this was a challenge, and I thought back to the two other times when I had encountered this problem—my kidney and breast surgeries.

The next Wednesday I stayed close to the phone, hoping the surgeon's secretary would call if the news was good. On Thursday morning, when I still had heard nothing, I reasoned that they either had not received the report or the news was bad and the doctor wanted to tell me personally.

Of course, there always was the chance that they had received news that morning and did not call because I had a 1:00 p.m. appointment. I tried to believe that.

As usual, Merv was going to meet me at the mall close to the surgeon's office and we would go together from there. As I drove to that mall, I chose to sing praise songs all the way even though I did not feel like it. It was a wise choice as those words gave me great encouragement and inner peace. I walked around the mall while waiting for Merv, but I had no interest whatsoever in anything I saw in the shop windows. My mind was already at the surgeon's office. When Merv arrived we went to the food court and ordered a large fries. That was forbidden food on my diet, but they were delicious. It reminded me of feeding a convict a big, delicious meal before executing him. Reluctantly we walked to the car, and soon we were entering the big medical building. I was really beginning to hate that place!

After a brief wait, I was called in and my first words to the surgeon were, "Well, what was it?" His answer, that it was the same as my shoulder lump, absolutely stunned me. Another metastasis of kidney cancer! Another death sentence! I went through the motions of taking off my sweater and he quickly removed the stitches. He then called Merv in, and I just shook my head. When Merv was told what it was, he immediately put his hand on mine, and I clung to it. The doctor read part of the lab report and slowly the horrendous words sank in.

I was scheduled to come back in a month, and a Cancer Clinic appointment to see the renal cell oncologist was also booked.

As we left the building, Merv and I were hurting badly, but I also felt relieved. For me, the waiting period is always worse than getting the news, even if it is bad.

I made a quick decision to go to Anita's boarding place, as I knew that she sometimes was there at noon. I prayed that I hadn't missed her. She was planning to phone me at

4:00 p.m. when her afternoon classes ended, but I needed to tell her personally.

When she answered the door she said, "Well?" and I told her what I had just learned. She looked so disappointed and put her arms around me. I tried to be positive, stressing that I was feeling healthy, and that the lump had been small, but we both knew that our family had once again taken many steps backward in the Valley. I said that I felt so guilty about putting the family through this again, and she replied, "Mom, it's not you. It's that silly little body of yours." We both managed a chuckle as my height (or lack of it) has been the source of many family jokes. We discussed the upcoming appointments, and after a couple more minutes and a couple more hugs it was time for me to leave. As I reached the door she said as emphatically as she could, "Mom, you *are* going to be at my wedding and you *are* going to see my kids!" I agreed and hurried out to my car so she wouldn't see the tears welling up in my eyes.

Ever since she was a very young teenager, Anita would poke me and whisper, "That's you and me in a couple of years," whenever we would see a young woman with a small child accompanied by a Grandma. I knew how important my being there would be for her.

I decided to sing more praise songs on the way home and I belted out "I Exalt Thee" almost at the top of my voice. I felt like Habakkuk who said long ago:

Though the fig tree does not bud
and there are no grapes on the vine
though the olive crop fails
and the fields produce no food
though there are no sheep in the pen
and no cattle in the stalls
YET WILL I REJOICE IN THE LORD
I WILL BE JOYFUL IN GOD MY SAVIOR
(Hab. 3:17-18)

I had a few lines of my own:
Though the lab reports are bad
and the prognosis dismal
though my days are numbered
and the cancer spreads
though all hope seems gone
and my heart is sad
YET WILL I REJOICE IN THE LORD!

When I arrived home I immediately made some phone calls. The school secretary needed to know that I would not be available until further notice. I made an appointment to see the holistic physician, hoping that he would prescribe more vitamins and supplements. When I phoned Dave, he could not hide his dismay. His voice sounded flat and all my comments of how well I was feeling and how small the lump was, could not change his frame of mind. Next I phoned an elder to get the prayer chain going on our behalf as I knew that this was one family that would be needing lots of prayer. By that night I had phoned all the friends and family that needed to know. Tomorrow would be a new day in the Valley of the Shadow of Cancer.

❧◦❧

Ever since our trip at Christmas, I had noticed that the area of my abdomen where my kidney had been removed, had been feeling uncomfortable. I had been especially aware of it the week that Merv and I had spent so much time sitting by the fire. I reminded myself that it always was uncomfortable when I sat for long periods of time or wore snug belts. Those things seemed to irritate the bowel that had looped itself as it filled in the space created by my surgery. Trying to sit in a comfortable position was impossible at times, and I could feel it with every step I took. Knowing that the muscle tissue on the rib cage had been cut to remove the last tumor, helped give me some peace of mind. Many weeks passed before that side felt normal again. Dozens of times I would think of many simple explanations for the discomfort. But always, in the back of my mind, I wondered if there was a large tumor there—another metastasis.

In spite of all of this, Merv and I were having a ball cooking all sorts of new recipes. He had bought a new cookbook by Dr. Paavo Airola, whose diet was similar to the one I had been advised to follow, so we decided to "go for it!" It was basically lots of whole grains, seeds and legumes, lots of vegetables—mostly raw, and some fruit. I felt extremely healthy (except for my side) and I lost eight pounds.

One day, as I brushed some lint off my sweater with my hand, I felt a rather large lump in the same breast that had the three cysts aspirated a few weeks earlier. It could easily be felt through my bra, turtleneck and sweater! I felt a choking panic rising in me as I explored my new finding very carefully. It was quite large—about the circumference of a quarter. It did not feel like a cyst. I knew that a tumor could not have developed that fast, so why didn't the surgeon feel this one when he had aspirated the cysts? A very horrifying thought started to develop in my mind. Maybe it was a tumor that had been hidden by those three cysts. I wish I had a switch on my mind that I could turn off when such thoughts begin to surface. I tried to convince myself that it might be a fibrous lump, so I decided to watch it carefully. I would show it to the surgeon at my next appointment in two weeks. Now, in addition to the recent metastasis, I had to deal with a side that continued to feel as if there was a large tumor below my ribs and a new breast lump that did not feel like a cyst. It took a lot of prayer that night before sleep finally came, giving much needed rest to my tortured mind and emotions.

When that lump felt exactly the same after a week of praying that it would disappear, my concerns increased. One morning, during my prayer time, I experienced for the first time in my life, a faint twinge of anger at God. I thought that coping with my kidney metastasis would have been enough, so it seemed inconceivable that a loving, caring Father would allow my side to feel as if there was a tumor there, and also allow that new breast lump to remain. How could He do this to me? Did He not know this was too much stress? I am well aware that many Christian counselors and pastors teach that anger at God is acceptable, even therapeutic, but I discovered that morning that it is not the answer for me. As I allowed the anger to rise within my spirit, I felt farther and farther from God. That was dismaying since I believed that He was the only source of my hope, peace and healing. I realized that I needed to be very near to Him, as a little child. As I repented of my rebellious spirit, I could once again feel the love of my Heavenly Father completely enfold me. Somehow there had to be some divine purpose for all of this, so I decided to let God be God, even though I did not understand. After all, my life (or death) was entirely in His hands, and He promised never to leave us or forsake us (Heb. 13:5b). As my faith increased, my anger dissipated. It was good to be back in the shadow of His wings once again (Ps. 17:8).

∽ 27 ∾

*F*ebruary was busy with many doctor's appointments. Merv and I saw the holistic medical doctor first. He was pleased at my decision to go all the way on the diet, and decided that I should take two new antioxidants in addition to the immune system boosters I was already taking. Once again we talked about the spiritual side of coping with this disease, agreeing that my future was entirely in God's hands. Nevertheless, we would do all we could to keep my body healthy until the end of the days God had allotted to me.

I asked him about juice fasting, as I had come across it many times in my recent reading. He cautioned me that a long juice fast could be very dangerous for me because I have only one kidney. The toxins that the body releases during a juice fast could damage my kidney, overworking it. I also asked him about (horror of horrors) enemas, as I had read several articles on that too. We soon decided that I was not ready to go that far!

He told us that we should get a book called *A Cancer Battle Plan* written by Anne E. Frähm and her husband David. Her breast cancer had spread to her shoulder, ribs, skull, pelvic bone and spine. But after surgery, cobalt, chemotherapy and a bone marrow transplant, she still had cancer and was sent home to die. She then turned to nutrition, exercise, detoxifiers and supplements, along with a lot of prayer. She beat cancer! The doctor told me that her actions and therapies had been more aggressive than mine. As soon as we got home, Merv phoned a Christian bookstore and was delighted to discover that they had the book. He would pick it up the next day.

By now my days were spent baking whole grain bread (no sugar or oil), chopping endless piles of vegetables, making kefir and my own whole grain pasta, taking long walks and spending lots of time in prayer. I was very busy, but also very contented.

✌◦✍

The night Merv brought the book home, we quickly ate, did the dishes and then I sat down to read. I was absolutely fascinated as I read *A Cancer Battle Plan*. I just couldn't put it down, and every few minutes I would say, "Merv, listen to this!" It was encouraging because I was already doing most of the things that she had done, but there was more. It involved what she called the E-word—enemas. There it was again! She also did a two-week juice fast, but I knew that was out for me. Even so, in spite of the E-word, I phoned the doctor early the next morning to inform him that I was ready to be as aggressive as the author was. Another appointment was set up. From reading that book, my attitude changed from thinking of controlling cancer to getting rid of it totally. A line from Anne Frähm's book: "Kick cancer's butt!"

The next evening as we were finishing the dishes, I asked Merv what time I should meet him at the mall the following day for my appointment with the renal cell oncologist. His reply made my heart sing. "You don't have to meet me anywhere because I'm taking the day off work." We decided that we would go into town early, do some shopping and errands and then have a bite to eat at a health food store that has a small cafe. It was the only place we could think of where I could eat without cheating on my diet (French fries were definitely not an option this time!).

I went to bed that night very happy and at peace, but I still had some concerns about the chest x-ray and blood work done at my last appointment in December. At one point I had considered phoning the oncologist for those test results, but I just didn't have enough courage to do that. I had told Merv and had secretly hoped he would phone, but I had completely forgotten that. Shortly after 3 a.m., I woke up in an absolute panic. The instant I woke up I had the thought that Merv had probably phoned the oncologist. The news was bad (cancer spread to the lungs), so he had decided not to tell me. Instead, he had taken the day off work so I wouldn't have to drive home alone after getting more devastating news.

As I lay there, I felt very cold as fear wound its icy tentacles around my whole being. I desperately wanted to know, but I decided to wait until morning. After all, if this was true, neither of us would get any more sleep, and I did not want to put Merv through that. I tried praying, but my terror increased. After a few minutes I just blurted out, "Merv did you phone the oncologist?" He said, "What?" in a voice that seemed to be coming from a thousand miles away. I asked him again, and this time he replied, "No, why?" He was beginning to wake up and this whole scene made absolutely no sense to him. I asked once again, "So you didn't phone the Cancer Clinic about those tests?" and he said he had not. I then explained what I had suspected, trying to hide my panic. He squeezed my arm, reassured me that he had not phoned, and soon his deep, even breathing told me he was asleep again. I lay awake the rest of the night. Even though this had all been in my imagination, it had been one of the most terrifying experiences I had encountered in the Valley. I prayed a lot and thanked God that I had been wrong. I was very glad when morning finally came, even though I would be getting those test results in a few hours.

≈≈≈

We had a great time shopping, marveling at how that tiny lump had changed our shopping habits during the past few weeks. I had always bought the groceries at an ordinary grocery store, but now our time at the regular store was very short. Our purchases there were limited to items like toiletries, detergent and cat food. The rest of the groceries were bought at a large fruit and vegetable store and at the health food store that has the little cafe.

We had a delightful lunch there. Merv had soup and I chose tabouleh (parsley and bulgur salad). That fit my diet, and having made it many times myself, I knew I would enjoy it. We chatted and laughed as we ate, and I thought that no one who saw us would have guessed that we had a very "heavy duty" appointment at the Cancer Clinic in half an hour.

As we drove to the hospital, I checked how I looked in the sun visor mirror. I discovered that the tabouleh had stuck between my teeth. I do not carry an extra toothbrush with me, so I hoped that the people in the cars beside us would not notice me picking little green specks from between my teeth with my fingernail!

When I entered the clinic's revolving door, I remembered how distraught and confused I had been seven weeks earlier, when I had left the hospital through that same door. At that time I was convinced I had breast cancer again, but instead I was returning with kidney cancer. Life in the Valley truly is unpredictable, and somehow that revolving door seems appropriate.

The first doctor asked whatever had happened, since all the tests at my last visit were perfectly normal. I certainly was very glad to hear that! She asked me many questions—all symptoms of the cancer spreading throughout my body—but I was able to answer "no" to all of them except the weight loss. I knew that she could see from my chart that I had lost about twelve pounds, so I explained that it was due to a change in my diet, not the cancer. I told her that I was eating lots of vegetables, whole grains, legumes, and no animal products whatsoever. When she asked me if I felt good eating like that, I once again realized that most oncologists have no idea about the connection between nutrition and cancer. It just did not dawn on her that I might have changed my diet to help fight my disease.

Next the examination began. She checked every square inch of my skin to see if there were any irregularities or lumps; there weren't. She felt my lymph nodes to see if she could find any swollen ones; she couldn't. Then she pounded my spine with her fist to see if it would hurt; it didn't, and she palpated my abdomen to see if there were any organ abnormalities; there weren't! I was beginning to enjoy this appointment after all. In the middle of the examination she stopped, looked very concerned, and said to me, "You must get really scared sometimes." I told her that most times I had peace, not fear, because many friends were praying for me. Then she asked if I believed in prayer, and I assured her I did. She said nothing.

When I was dressed again, Merv was called in and the doctor returned with the renal cell oncologist whom I had seen two years earlier. She immediately joked about having done such a good job of getting rid of me the last time, that I had stayed away for two years. It was obvious that she was delighted that I was looking and feeling so well. She then got serious and commented that I had a very slow progressing kidney cancer, and that she would like the rest of the tests to be done, "so we can stage you and see how far along you are." I guess that's the polite way of saying that she wanted to know how long until I die. I noticed that she said nothing about the one to two per cent chance of survival. She was certainly treating it as terminal.

The bone scan was the first test she suggested, and once again I refused it. She agreed that they could not do anything for me if they found it in my bones, but if they found "hot spots" (sites of cancer in the bones), they could tell me where they were so I could protect that part of my body. That might prevent a bone fracture. I did not budge, so she told the other doctor to write "refused" beside that test.

I consented to have the ultrasound and blood work which would determine the state and function of my organs. The blood work could be done immediately on site, but I would have to wait four weeks for the ultrasound. I had hoped to have a shorter wait, but even so, I was a very happy, thankful person as I left the Cancer Clinic and went on to the blood lab.

The technician there seemed to be having trouble withdrawing my blood, and as she was working with the syringe in my arm, she asked if I had been in a hot place. I thought it might be harder to draw blood when one was overheated, so I replied, "I've been in this hospital for over an hour." She just cracked up with laughter and explained that she meant a holiday in the tropics because of my tan. We both laughed when I told her about my beta carotene tan.

❧❧

A week later I had my appointment with the surgeon. He wanted to check the incision and the area around it to see that there was no recurrence of the tumor. I thought that all was well in that area, but of course, there was that new breast lump for him to check.

As I walked around the mall waiting to meet Merv, I noticed that the new colors for spring were my favorites— pinks, light blues and greens. The sweaters were lovely. I thought I should buy one to cheer myself up, but emotionally I couldn't handle that. My appointment would have to come first. Merv came, and once again we headed for that medical building which fills me with foreboding thoughts and emotions whenever I enter it.

Soon I was called into the examination room, and how I wished there was only the incision to be checked. The surgeon examined it and was very pleased. Then, with overwhelming fear, I showed him the lump in my breast. To my relief, he felt it briefly, announced that it had to be a cyst, and proceeded to aspirate it. Thank you Lord!! I couldn't understand why it felt so different from the other cysts. The doctor told me that sometimes cysts have a thicker membrane, and therefore feel different. I left that little room with a huge smile on my face. It was so fantastic to be given good news for a change. I joked with the secretary and Merv, and they too entered into my joy. I noticed that no one else was smiling. Those patients were still awaiting *their* turn to hear *their* news. But I was rejoicing. It is very important for us in the Valley to make the most of all our little victories, and this was my day to celebrate. In three weeks I would have my ultrasound and then *I* would be sitting, waiting and wondering.

❧

The next day was another day of unbelievable joy. Early in the morning I received a call from the Cancer Clinic, reporting "perfectly normal" results from the biochemical blood work. That news made me more convinced than ever that with prayer, a strict vegetarian diet, supplements, exercise and bowel cleansing, I maybe *could* "kick cancer's butt."

I had a good appointment with the holistic doctor, and was thrilled to report to him all the recent good news. He gave me a large container of metabolic detoxification powder along with instructions, daily schedules and recipes, for a very restrictive rotation diet. The E-word did not turn out to be as bad as I had thought. As I was not juice fasting, enemas only twice a week, instead of twice a day, would suffice.

I had thought that any drugstore would sell enema kits (the kind with the tube attached to a reservoir that looks like a small hot water bottle). When Merv insisted that I phone a pharmacy before going into town later that week, I thought he was being ridiculous. I soon realized that his suggestion was a very good one. It took many calls before I finally found a store that sold that kind of kit. The rest all said they could order one, but I needed it the next day, as I had already started the detoxification program.

I tried the E-procedure the next afternoon. I read and reread the instructions, and I almost talked myself out of the need to do it. I was to have a three stage enema—one liter (quart) of lukewarm water each time. The charcoal powder that had to be added to the water turned everything black. Merv helped me get set up and things proceeded very well. I couldn't feel any cramping or discomfort which the instructions had warned about. When I thought the bag should be empty I called Merv to check. He looked into the bag, and informed me that it was still full. A problem in the nozzle had prevented any of the water from flowing into my bowel. No wonder I had no discomfort!

We corrected the situation, and this time it worked. By the time I had taken in, held and expelled three successive liters, I felt like a pro. I kidded Merv that we might have to redecorate the bathroom, as the charcoal black water had not been confined, as I had hoped, to only the toilet bowl and garbage bag on which I had lain. I guess I needed more practice! By the time I had taken a shower and had everything cleaned up and in order in the bathroom, an hour and a half had elapsed. I really hoped that it had not been time wasted, but I was willing to do even this to increase my possibilities of getting rid of this disease once and for all.

One day I noticed that every coffee table, end table and night table in our house had at least one book on it with the word cancer or nutrition in its title. We certainly were doing our homework.

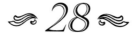

I had begun to ask God what He wanted me to do since I had quit teaching, on the advice of my doctors. One morning, during my prayer time, I felt very strongly that He was asking me to start a support group for women battling cancer. As I thought and prayed about this, I was excited. Maybe all I had gone through could benefit others. I decided to call the group CANSURVIVE—*Days of Encouragement.* The scripture that came to mind was Isaiah 41:10:

So do not fear for I am with you;
do not be dismayed, for I am your God.
I will strengthen you and help you;
I will uphold you with my righteous right hand.

It was wonderful to be able to plan for the future again.

≈ 28 ≈

*H*alfway through the detoxification program, I had the ultrasound to check my organs. It was very uneventful and took less than half an hour. The technician was quite pleasant, and even though she didn't say that all was well, I certainly had that feeling as I left the lab.

On the morning of my Cancer Clinic appointment to find out those results, Merv and I prayed together. We asked God to help us live in the knowledge that He is in control. We resolved not to let the doctors take charge of our lives by their information; instead, we would take God's word as our authority and comfort. Little did we know how relevant that was.

I actually had two appointments—first with the renal cell specialist, and then with the breast cancer specialist. We waited well over an hour until my name was finally called. To say that we were not tense would be stretching the truth because the results of that ultrasound were crucial. Merv came into the examining room with me, and again we had to wait. Finally my oncologist came in with my file and started reading the ultrasound report. She said there were several enlarged lymph nodes around my pancreas. My heart sank, and I managed to say, "That isn't good, is it?" She replied, "No."

The thought of the ultrasound showing the spread of kidney cancer into my lymph system had never crossed my mind. When I asked if those nodes could be surgically removed, the doctor said it would be pointless. I asked about my organs, and as she read on, we learned that they were normal. That encouraged me, but it did not seem to be important to the doctor. I said that I knew that not much could be done, and she agreed, but there were some options to consider.

Apparently, some people at this advanced stage travel to the United States to have a very expensive therapy using Interleukin-2. This is effective for only twenty-five per cent, but she emphasized that, for those patients, it was very beneficial. When I asked how much longer they lived, the oncologist said two years at the most. I made some quick mental calculations: a wait of several months, many months of feeling ill during and after the treatment, a few months of good health, followed by the return of the illness and declining health until I would die. To go deep into debt for that seemed ludicrous, so I said I was not interested.

Next, she offered chemotherapy. I informed her that I knew it was ineffective for kidney cancer and she agreed. When she went on to say that some patients become desperate enough to try it anyway, I replied that I wasn't that desperate.

Another option was experimental chemotherapy drugs, which I quickly refused. I was feeling perfectly healthy, and I knew that if I went that route I would suffer tremendously.

I was then told that the only thing left was to have an ultrasound and consultation every two months to monitor the stages of the disease. I reminded her that I had been told several times in the past that my cancer was a very slow progressing one, and she agreed. She said that even taking that into consideration, the very most I could expect of anything resembling health was six months! I realized that was a politically correct way of saying that in six months I would either be dead or dying. My world collapsed!! I looked at Merv, and the emotional trauma we both felt seemed to be tangible in that small room.

The oncologist went on to say that I would develop back pain because of the location of those lymph nodes. That added to my despair because I had felt some discomfort in my back for several weeks. I had planned to have my chiropractor check it sometime. When I showed her the location of the slight pain, she confirmed that it was exactly where she expected it to be.

I wanted to cry, but couldn't. The overwhelming emotions of fear, devastation and utter hopelessness were beyond tears.

My appointment with the breast cancer specialist was next, but I knew I couldn't deal with that. The oncologist said she would cancel it for me, saying, "I'm sorry," as she left. Merv and I just sat there. I wondered if I would ever have a normal day again, when death was not foremost on my mind. I resigned myself to the fact that I could not finish this book, nor could I start the support group.

⋙⋘

Scripture says, "Where there is no vision, the people perish" Pr. 29:18 (KJV). I had no vision left; I was perishing!

⋙⋘

We left in silence, picked up my appointment card, and went out that revolving door once again.

Merv suggested that we leave my car at the mall and go directly to share our devastation with Alf and Christa. We had told them that we would let them know, but they were expecting good news. After all, I was feeling one hundred per cent healthy.

When they saw our faces, they realized that something awful had happened. After hugs and a brief version of what had just transpired, I started to cry, and we all went into the living room to pray. They interceded for me while I wept. After about twenty minutes of intense prayer to the only One who could intervene and change the situation, I felt peace and hope rising within me. With great determination, I wiped my eyes and said, "I *can* finish my book and I *can* start my group!" Obviously God had known all along, and I knew that the peace and hope I was beginning to feel in my spirit once again was from Him.

⋙⋘

When they saw the sudden change in my demeanor, Christa said, "We were praying for a miracle and we're seeing one before our eyes." I joined them as they thanked God and praised Him for His love and mercy.

A Bible verse about not fearing bad news kept coming to my mind, but I couldn't find it in their Bible. Alf checked his concordance program on his computer and soon found it. "He will have no fear of bad news; his heart is steadfast, trusting in the Lord. His heart is secure; he will have no fear: in the end he will look in triumph on his foes" (Ps. 12:7-8). I certainly had received bad news, but this assured me that I need not fear. Christa and I discussed that concept while Merv and Alf got my car.

As we left their home, I felt ready once again to face the future. After all, I still had some living to do before my death. We would have to live by faith, not by sight (2 Cor. 5:7).

❧ 29 ❧

When we arrived home, several phone calls had to be made. Merv and I decided we would not tell the kids about the six month prognosis until after their final exams. They had enough stress. Because of our "secret," we could not put it on the prayer chain at church as the kids would have found out.

I phoned a few couples from church, told them the situation, asked for their prayers and swore them to secrecy. Even though those dear friends were absolutely shocked, and I could tell from their trembling voices how upset they were, those calls were the easy ones. The hardest would be to the family.

My brother just kept saying, "No, it can't be." I told him about the back pain which confirmed the prognosis. He and his wife had a difficult struggle in accepting that news.

I was unable to reach my sister until late that night. She, too, was absolutely stunned, and we talked for a very long time. That was one evening when long distance telephone charges were not important. How I wished we didn't live so far apart.

When I finally slumped into bed, I was exhausted, but sleep seemed to be very far away. Merv and I prayed together, and even though I had peace, the events of the day had left me emotionally drained. March 16, 1995, was a day we would never forget.

I awakened many times during that restless night. The thought that I had nothing to wear in the casket kept haunting me. I am definitely a jeans and dress pants person, and as I mentally went through my wardrobe, I realized that I had nothing suitable. I didn't think I should buy a dress in which to be buried (I'm much too frugal for that!), so I wondered what I would do. I finally decided to buy a new dress for a wedding in May, at which Anita would be a bridesmaid. That solved my problem. I'd buy a dress with long sleeves, suitable for any time of the year. I thought that long sleeves would be appropriate, as most cancer victims lose lots of weight before dying. My arms would look scrawny in short sleeves. (Be still, my prideful heart!)

When I awoke at 5:00 a.m., I realized that what I feared most was the ultrasound and the consultation which the oncologist had scheduled. I decided that I did not have to go through with that. After all, if there was nothing that could be done, why put myself through that stress? I would return to that oncologist if the symptoms became a problem, but not before. When Merv awoke, I told him about my decision. His answer was very wise. He agreed that the choice was mine, but he strongly suggested that I not cancel the appointments until the week before the scheduled time. That would leave room to change my mind. I felt as if a great burden had been lifted from me.

Since we both were wide awake after a restless night, we took our first of many early morning walks along the beach. We drew strength from each other and from God as we walked hand in hand, hardly saying a word. I thought back to our marriage vows: "In sickness and health" and "'til death do us part." I once again realized how difficult these situations are for the spouse. When I died I would be with the Lord, but Merv would become a widower, having lost his companion of over twenty-seven years.

Later that morning I made appointments with the chiropractor and holistic physician. I also phoned both kids and prayed a lot before making those calls. I asked God to camouflage any fear or tension that they might detect in my voice. I told each of them the truth: there was no cancer in my organs (I really stressed that), but some lymph nodes needed to be checked in a few months. I did not say anything about the six-month prognosis. I continued to talk about finishing this book and preparing the brochures for CanSurvive. By God's grace, neither suspected anything.

That entire day I was very aware of my back. It was as though all my thoughts were being focused on that area of my body. Finally, I had trouble distinguishing between real or imaginary pain. I couldn't wait to get to the chiropractor to find out the cause. I spent most of the day praying, reading the Bible and listening to my "comfort" tapes.

❧❧

The next day I was still very conscious of my back, but in spite of that, I had peace. After lunch I lay down with my small tape player, and all at once I began to wonder how I would say good-bye to my family. All I could think of was to tell the kids, "I would have been a good Grandma." Extreme sadness enveloped my whole being, and I began to cry inconsolably. Even when I got up and walked around, the tears kept coming. The thought of saying good-bye to Merv and the kids, in a little more than six months, was unthinkable. After a long time of sobbing, the telephone rang. I was tempted to just leave it, but decided to answer it anyway. I cleared my throat and practiced talking as I walked to the phone. I did not want the caller to guess from my voice that I had been crying. In a very controlled manner, I answered the phone, and Anita said, "Hi, Mom! What are you doing?" Her cheerful voice was like a soothing salve on an open wound. We talked very briefly as she just wanted the name of my new vegetarian cookbook. By the time I hung up, my sadness had entirely left. It was as if God had used that phone call to say, "You're not saying good-bye today." The rest of the day was filled with deep joy and an abiding trust that God was in control. The fact that I might be dying in six months was not in my "box for today."

When I went to the chiropractor, I was relieved that he found a misalignment in my lower back—the probable cause of my pain. He adjusted it and told me to come back in a few days.

That night Merv massaged my back and continued to do so each evening for several weeks. After two more chiropractic adjustments my back problem was gone, so I knew that the lymph nodes were not the cause. That was very encouraging!

In the meantime, Anita suggested that we should go shopping for my dress for the wedding. She did not notice that I tried on only those with long sleeves. We found a beautiful light green, two piece outfit. By then I had lost about fifteen pounds, so we both thought it looked excellent.

Usually when I buy clothing, I model them for Merv when I get home, but I just couldn't. When I put the dress on three days later, I realized that I couldn't keep it. To me it was a dress in which to be buried, and I hated it. It was returned to the store the next day. Several weeks later Merv and I went shopping and I bought one with *short* sleeves. No more casket dresses for me!

My appointment with the holistic physician finally came, and he was shocked when I told him my news. He was adamant that no one can determine the cause of swollen lymph nodes from an ultrasound alone. Only a biopsy could tell what was causing the enlargement. Since I had been on the metabolic detoxification program at the time of the ultrasound, that could perhaps have been the cause of the swelling. He admitted that it was very possible that I did have kidney cancer in those nodes, but he also reminded me that I had very successfully battled that cancer for well over six years. He thought that the mention of six months was like a curse, and cautioned me to completely reject it because it was a prognosis based on insufficient evidence.

We again discussed the whole issue that God was the One to decide. The doctor prescribed homeopathic drops, which are specifically used to reduce the swelling of lymph nodes. I felt like a convict on death row who had been given a reprieve. Merv had been unable to come with me, so that night I eagerly told him all the doctor had said.

I phoned my brother and sister to tell them that there might be some hope after all.

❧ 30 ❧

*T*he following weeks were filled with much joy and peace. I continued to keep all animal products out of my diet, and with the purchase of several new vegetarian cookbooks, Merv and I had lots of fun trying out new recipes. Both the doctor and I thought that my weight loss (now twenty pounds) was due to my restrictive diet and long daily walk. I had no health complaints whatsoever, and Merv and I were very thankful for each day.

After much stalling, I finally made an appointment with my family doctor for my yearly checkup. I had completely forgotten it the previous year, so this was very important, even though I cringed at the thought of seeing another doctor.

When I arrived, my doctor, who had not seen me for two years, remarked that I looked very well. Even though she had received the report from the Cancer Clinic, she was very shocked when I told her that I was not planning to die in the next few months. She checked the report when I explained what I meant, and immediately noted that she did not see a biopsy report on the lymph nodes. It was soon evident that she felt the same as the holistic physician—without a biopsy, no one could determine the cause of the swelling.

After she had completed the Pap test, she told me that she had seen something on my cervix. She said it did not look like cancer, so the worst it could be was dysplasia (pre-cancerous cells), which is very easy to treat. She also told me that an appointment with a specialist would be arranged, even if the results were negative. That was a precautionary measure due to my medical history.

I certainly wasn't thrilled about her discovery, but was determined to leave it in God's hands. After much prayer, I did not worry at all. In less than a week I received the results. My blood pressure shot sky high when I heard the nurse's voice, but she had good news. There were no malignant cells; only some inflammatory cells were evident. She also gave me the date of my appointment with the specialist. When I discovered that the specialist, instead of being a gynecologist as I had assumed, was really a gynecological *oncologist*, I was very upset. My joy at hearing the negative results was replaced by terror and panic. I thought back to Bea again. "It never ends." It took a lot of prayer and talking to Merv that night to get back on track again.

≈⊷

The appointment with the gynecological oncologist was more than a week away, so I tried even harder to stay in my "box for today."

When that day finally arrived, Merv went with me, and both of us were dealing with very fragile emotions. It had been only five weeks earlier that we had been told about the six months, and now we were wondering if I had another cancer.

When the specialist examined me, she said that the lesion did not look like cancer. Then she proceeded to do another Pap test, as well as a biopsy. I felt no pain or discomfort, and soon some packing was put into place to stop any bleeding. The doctor once again said that it did not look like cancer, so even if the report did come back positive, the malignant cells would be at a very early stage and, therefore, quite treatable. I was given a date and time, two and a half weeks away, to call her office for the results. I felt very vulnerable as we left the building, but I was happy that I was to phone for the results. That was much better than waiting to hear from them, and panicking every time the phone rang.

❧❧

By now it was time for me to cancel the ultrasound and consultation with the kidney cancer specialist. I did that with much joy and confidence, as I had discussed my decision with several doctors. With much apprehension, I kept the appointment with the breast cancer specialist. The fluctuating lump seemed to have stabilized and was not changing anymore. I convinced myself that it felt like a cyst, so I decided to have the surgeon check it before going to the clinic.

The week starting May 7 was a week to remember. My appointment with the surgeon was on Tuesday. On Thursday I was to see the breast cancer specialist at the Cancer Clinic, and on Friday morning I was to phone the Dysplasia Clinic to find out whether or not I had cervical cancer. Merv and I concluded that if we would get through that week, we could probably deal with anything the future had to offer.

On Tuesday, when I told the surgeon about the six months, he was very concerned. He said the same as the other doctors—without a biopsy, no one could say for sure that cancer was causing the lymph node swelling. He was shocked that a doctor would tell me that I had no more than six months of anything resembling health, when all the other tests were normal. I was very encouraged by his kind, supportive words, and when he was able to aspirate the lump, I was absolutely delighted. It was a cyst! (One down—two to go!)

On Thursday I met with a new breast cancer doctor, and

for the first time an oncologist listened, with interest, as I told him what I was doing to fight my disease. He had seen the report on the kidney cancer and was amazed at how well I looked and how emotionally together I appeared to be. I told him about all the prayer and everything the holistic physician had recommended. He was fascinated, and finally told me to continue everything because it obviously was working. He checked my breasts and everything was normal. I told him I would not be seeing the kidney oncologist regularly, because I doubted that a doctor who had put a time limit on my health (and therefore my life) could be of much help. He wished me well and told me to come back in six months. He also advised me to continue seeing the holistic doctor. I was so pleased that he had been interested enough to ask what I was doing. It had been a very uplifting appointment. (Two down—one to go!)

The next morning I made the phone call to the Dysplasia Clinic at 9:01 a.m. The line was already busy and continued to be busy for the next half hour. Obviously, I was not the only person who was anxious to get her test results. Finally, I got through and the news was fantastic—no malignant cells! I was told to have another Pap test in six months, and was reassured that I did not have cervical cancer. (Three down—none to go!)

I called Merv and we rejoiced on the phone. We arranged to take Alf and Christa to an organic vegetarian restaurant to celebrate. We thanked God that the week was over and that all the news had been excellent.

That evening during the meal, a magnificent double rainbow appeared. It was so spectacular that the diners who did not have window seats came over to look. Many remarked that they had never seen one that brilliant. As we watched the rainbow, we noticed some birds flying in front of it. The rest of the sky was very dark blue, and as the sun shone on the birds, they looked like pure gold. It was an awesome sight. I thought of the first rainbow, and how God's promises are as true now as then. During that "heavy duty" week we had experienced His promises of peace first hand. We had a wonderful time and went home feeling very secure in God's hands.

∾∾

In the weeks that followed, I continued my morning walks, reveling in the beauty of spring. After their exams, I told the kids about the six-month prognosis (which by then was four months), and both accepted the news very well. I was looking and feeling one hundred per cent healthy, so it was easier for them to hope it was a misdiagnosis.

I continued to make plans for my CANSURVIVE support group. I needed to find lots of new vegetarian recipes, as I would be providing breakfast and lunch. I visited many pastors in the area and left my brochures with them. They all were very pleased that there was someone to whom they could refer parishioners suffering from cancer. I felt very strongly that cancer patients needed to know the benefits of prayer, diet, exercise and a positive outlook.

Summer '95 was a wonderful time for our whole family. The weather was great and I had no medical appointments. The 16th day of each month required a little celebration because it reminded us that one more month of my death sentence had passed without any sign of illness. By fall, my regular checkups began again, and we were relieved that my follow-up six-month Pap test was clear.

At present, my surgeon and I are watching a small lump that has developed near my last incision. Since it might be scar tissue, instead of a metastasis, we have decided to postpone surgery until it is large enough to remove with local anesthetic. We feel that it is in my best interest to protect my body from more general anesthetic. So obviously, living in my "box for today" is still very important, especially since Christmas (with its memories of my other crises) is just around the corner.

*A*s I come to the end of this book, I know that it is not the end of the story. I have been in the Valley for many years now, and our family life has changed. Dave has graduated with an honors degree in Geology and is presently doing post-graduate studies in Nova Scotia. Anita has graduated from Medical Office Administration, as well as her Children's Literature correspondence course, and is continuing her studies. My mother is in a special care unit for Alzheimer and dementia patients. Merv and I are enjoying our empty nester status. He still has the same job, and my CANSURVIVE—*Days of Encouragement* support group has become a telephone ministry. Most of the women who have contacted me are on chemotherapy, and therefore are usually too ill to come to my house. We all benefit from the information we share in our conversations, and commit ourselves to praying daily for each other.

Writing this book has been difficult for both Anita and me. She typed it on her computer, and together we edited it. There were times when we had to stop because the memories were overwhelming. At times Anita would be shocked because she and Dave had been unaware of many of the minor crises (false alarms). One day we had a real scare. I was just dictating a sentence about the need for one of my surgeries. While we were reliving the tensions of that moment, the phone rang. It was the doctor who had performed that surgery, with the results of my last mammogram. When I heard his voice I almost fainted. He had good news, but the timing of the call was awful. After the initial shock, Anita and I had a good laugh and continued.

Six and a half years have passed since the removal of my kidney and spleen, four years since my breast cancer, three years since my first metastasis and almost a year since my last. It is nine months since I was given what I call my "six-month death sentence." According to the statistics, I should not be alive, but even if I am in that one to two per cent who do survive, I'll have several more years in the Valley. In fact, it is my opinion that one never quite gets out of it. The memories and physical scars remain. Even so, I am feeling perfectly healthy, have lots of energy and enjoy every day to the fullest.

Since entering the Valley I have gone from a 45-year-old to a 52-year-old who is experiencing the hormonal changes typical of that age. I do not attempt to comprehend why God has spared me. I am well aware that since I first had cancer, hundreds of thousands of others have died from it. I thank God for His mercy and healing, and pray that I may always glorify Him in my life. I continue to put into practice what I believe will help fight this disease. I faithfully take all the vitamins, supplements, antioxidants, etc., and my diet is still vegetarian. We buy as much organic produce as our budget allows. I also avoid all processed foods and those containing white flour, sugar, refined oils and chemicals. Herbal teas, freshly made fruit and vegetable juices and lots of water have totally replaced coffee and regular tea. I am also experimenting with the proper combining of foods. I try to walk briskly for an hour each day, and getting enough sleep is a must. As always, I spend regular time with the Lord every morning, and many people continue to pray for me daily.

❦

It is my prayer that those who read my story will see how faithful God has always been to our family and will know that His love and mercy are promised to their family too. Nevertheless, no one should expect Him to do for them exactly what He has done for me. In each of my struggles, He has worked very differently. Yes, there have been many times of fear, sadness and absolute hopelessness, but by His grace they have been short. Only time will tell what my prognosis really is, but with Him I can face the future, confident in His love. In the meantime I will continue to walk with my family, knowing that my life is entirely in His hands. Lamentations 3:22-23 says:

Because of the Lord's great love
we are not consumed
for His compassions never fail.
They are new every morning;
Great is Your faithfulness.

Those words best describe my continuing journey in the Valley of the Shadow of Cancer.

Publishers Note—March 1996

At the time of publication, Eleanor Bouwman has had surgery for the removal of the lump on her rib cage. It proved to be a metastasis of kidney cancer, a recurrence of the previous tumor at that site. Subsequent test results were excellent, revealing that those lymph nodes which had prompted her "six-month death sentence" given a year ago are now normal. She continues to feel one hundred per cent healthy.

Appendix

Hints for Cancer Warriors

The following tips have helped me and I share them with you.

1. I always spend quality time with the Lord in the early morning. This sets the tone for the day. *Morning by morning, O Lord, You hear my voice...*(Ps. 5:3a). *But I cry to You for help, O Lord; in the morning my prayer comes before You* (Ps. 88:13).

2. I study the scriptures daily, and meditate on those verses which give me hope and comfort. *Your word is a lamp unto my feet and a light unto my path* (Ps.119 :105).

3. When I first had cancer, I came to terms with dying. That has made my subsequent crises much less frightening. *Where, O death is your victory? Where, O death is your sting?* (1Cor. 15:55). *For me to live is Christ and to die is gain* (Phil. 1:21).

4. I attend special healing services, only when I feel the Holy Spirit prompting me. To do otherwise would lead to a frantic path of frustration, disappointment, and much confusion. *Is any one of you sick? He should call the elders of the church to pray over him and anoint him with oil in the name of the Lord* (James 5:14). *Man's days are determined; You have decreed the number of his months and have set limits he cannot exceed* (Job 14:5).

5. I always keep in mind that God, not the doctors, has the final say in my future. *All the days ordained for me were written in Your book before one of them came to be* (Ps. 139:16b).

6. I have a few close friends who will pray for me, as well as

keep my confidential concerns to themselves. Even though our church has a prayer chain, there have been some minor or personal problems that not everyone needed to know. *A gossip betrays a confidence, but a trustworthy man keeps a secret* (Prov. 11:13).

7. Although we have always been very honest with our children, we usually have chosen not to tell them our suspicions or concerns until they have been confirmed by a doctor.

8. When I wait for my turn in a doctor's office or clinic, I pray instead of reading the outdated magazines. This focuses my mind on God and His peace, rather than on my fears. *Thou wilt keep him in perfect peace, whose mind is stayed on Thee; because he trusteth in Thee* (Is. 26:3 KJV).

9. We have bought a very large medical encyclopedia. If we had had it in the beginning, I would have known immediately that hypernephroma is another name for kidney cancer. Now I read up on any new condition or procedure as soon as I get home from my appointments.

10. Having a holistic medical doctor and chiropractor, in addition to the oncologists, has been a tremendous blessing. Each has studied a different approach to medicine, and I continue to benefit from all of them.

11. Living in my "box for today" makes the period of waiting for test results much less tense. It takes self discipline to stay in that box, but with prayer it is possible and very crucial to the enjoyment of life. *Therefore, do not worry about tomorrow, for tomorrow will worry about itself. Each day has enough trouble of its own* (Matt. 6:34). *Who of you by worrying can add a single hour to his life?* (Matt. 6:27).

12. Sticking to my diet is very challenging, but I am encouraged by actively fighting cancer in this way. (I have discov-

ered that potluck affairs are much more enjoyable when I take a main course dish as well as a salad and dessert that fit my diet.)

13. A good sense of humor has helped me through some very trying circumstances. *A cheerful heart is good medicine, but a crushed spirit dries up the bones* (Prov. 17:22).

14. I do not try to be my own doctor. I never take vitamins or supplements, etc., without getting my doctor's approval, since taking large amounts of some of those substances can have serious side effects.

15. We have bought many books dealing with the relationship between nutrition and disease, and while they don't agree on every point, I pick out that which sounds best for my situation and check it out with my doctor. *Listen to advice and accept instruction, and in the end you will be wise* (Prov. 19:20).

16. Reading books by other cancer patients who have survived has been very encouraging for both Merv and me. I highly recommend this, but once again, I do not try their suggestions without my doctor's approval.

17. When I find that the diet restrictions, the vitamin and supplement regime (including the wretched-tasting vitamin C and green barley powders), enemas, and my daily walks, are becoming a burden, I reread Anne Frähm's book, *A Cancer Battle Plan*. This gives me the inspiration to continue.

18. I am learning to make the most of every day, trying to live by Saint Paul's admonition: *Be joyful always; pray continually; give thanks in all circumstances, for this is God's will for you in Christ Jesus* (1 Thes. 5:16-18).